A CANCER SURVIVAL GUIDE

FEARLESS HEALING

AMEENA MEER

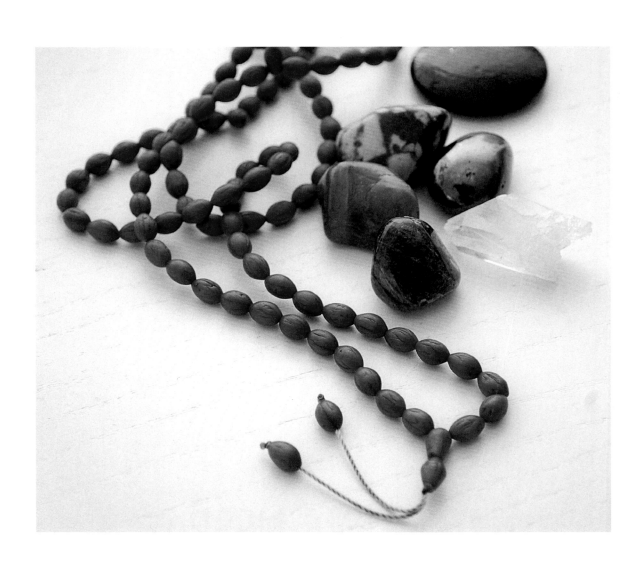

WHENEVER YOU ARE
CONFRONTED
WITH AN OPPONENT,
CONQUER HIM
WITH LOVE.

- GANDHI

Book design: Take Out Media
Cover images: Gabriel Eid
Interior photographs: Sasha Douglas-Nares
Illustration: Baris Hasirci
Calligraphy: Thich Nhat Hanh

Library of Congress Control Number: 2017930712
Fearless Healing, Brooklyn, NEW YORK

Disclaimer (required for legal reasons)

The content of this book is for general informational purposes only. It is not meant to be used, nor should it be used, to diagnose or treat any medical condition or to replace the services of your physician or other health care provider. The advice and strategies contained in the book may not be suitable for all readers. Please consult your health care provider for any questions that you may have about your own medical situation. Neither the author, publisher, IIN nor any of their employees or representatives guarantees the accuracy of information in this book or its usefulness to a particular reader, nor are they responsible for any damages or negative consequences that may result from any treatment, action taken, or inaction by any person reading or following the information in this book.

To contact the author, visit **www.Fearlesshealing.net**

ISBN 978-0998582191

Printed in the United States of America

to Sasha, Zarina and Jahanara

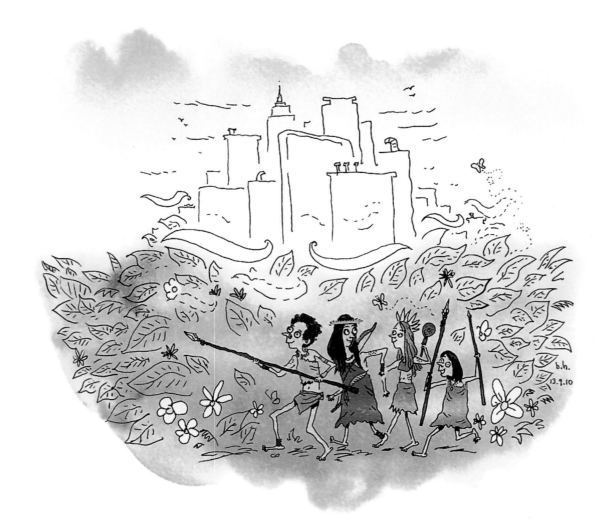

An Introduction: Why I Am Writing This

In 2012, amongst Americans of both genders and all races, there was a 40% chance of developing cancer in their lifetimes and, for women, a 19% chance of dying of it (according the National Institutes of Cancer's latest report. This number has not gone down. That means, amongst five of your friends, chances are, two will develop cancer. That is a big number. Depending on your age, socio-economic and/or genetic group, the number may be even higher.

I am a liberal, a Muslim, and was a single mother raising three teenaged girls in New York City. I may be nothing like you. But I was one of the 800,000 new cancer cases of 2009. In this, we are all together.

There is no "What to Expect When You're Not Expecting It" of cancer. No "Cancer for Dummies." People hush it up. It can feel like a failing grade, a punishment for bad lifestyle habits or bad behavior. Just when we need most to talk about it, we don't. We hide it or try and erase it.

First, I called both the illness and the book the c-word because people are terrified of it. Because it's like the bubonic plague. You don't even want to say it around people because they see it as such a downer. It's bad. It's evil. Way scarier than the other c-word. My mother told me to take down all the pictures of myself when I was bald on my Facebook account. But I am proud of it. Every picture is evidence of my climb up Mount Everest. I was laughing and enjoying the people around me the whole way. (I had dark moments, too, but wouldn't anyone? I'm just a regular person.)

Then I changed it to Fearless Healing. Because hearing the c-word can frighten you and it's your job to take the wheel and get your wellbeing under control. The c-word is the threat, not the reaction.

Once you face your healing as well as your fear, you own it.

In my mind, owning your health is the key to healing it. It means taking responsibility for your body and your soul. It doesn't mean guilt or blame, it means picking up the pieces and building something powerful.

No one wants to get cancer. Cancer is a furious uprising in your body. Like so many other disasters, it takes over your life and the lives of the people around you. Unlike a broken arm or the flu, however, its course is unpredictable even by doctors with decades of experience. When you come out the other end, you will find yourself transformed, psychically and physically. If nothing else, cancer is a trial by fire.

While skydivers, bungee-jumpers, firewalkers, speakers-in-tongues, born-agains of all stripes and religions, devotees of the Landmark Forum or AA say that you will be forever changed by the experience—the reality is, almost nothing will uproot you like cancer. Most people, after contracting cancer, think differently about every breath and every sunrise. Yes, I know a couple of people who stayed the same, but they didn't last long.

So here is my promise to you: This too will pass. You will come out the other end. It will not be the way you expect or the way you want it, but you will come out. It won't be easy or fun. It will force you to work like crazy. You, and everyone around you, will be strengthened by the process. Illness might just heal your life.

The truth of it is this: I was relieved to have cancer. I believe I chose it unconsciously. I knew I had cancer a couple of weeks before I was diagnosed. I mean, I didn't know empirically, but I knew it intuitively. I was really sick and weak and tired and the word "cancer" popped into my head. So I knew.

It was a particularly painful moment in my life. After a successful career, I hadn't had much work in months. I had gone through all of my savings. I lost my apartment, I was forced to sell my designer clothes and my furniture. I begged my exhusbands to help my kids stay in the apartment until the end of the school year. Instead, they sent me an email—together—suggesting the children might benefit from learning about hardship.

From there, we slipped from the frying pan into the fire. I moved apartments more or less by myself, with friends and a bunch of college students with shopping carts and old strollers. I was in and out of housing court. I hired a lawyer. I maxed out every credit card they would still give me to put in a second bathroom and some kitchen cabinets from IKEA. I sold my expensive handbags and my inherited midcentury modern furniture and we ate the proceeds. While I was able to keep my kids in the apartment until June, and eventually, in the same neighborhood, I did so at the expense of my physical and psychological wellbeing. My youngest kid got pulled out of 3rd grade and had to sit in the principal's office all day because I hadn't paid the school fees, one of my exhusbands told me I was exaggerating. Rats ate through the wiring of my car. Ice crashed through my skylights showering the rooms in broken glass, the whole place flooded repeatedly. One of my exhusbands sued ME for emotional distress. The lawyer didn't show up in housing court, instead he sent crazy emails and I lost by default. People said, "Well, at least things can't get worse!"

It turned out that things got worse. As a friend of mine pointed out, "You'd been through A LOT. Something had to give."

When I was diagnosed, I was at my lowest point. Though terrified, I felt released. I thought that having cancer would force everyone to be kinder to me. That people who had been horrid to me would be sorry and remember that I had some good points. I thought I'd be in a hospital room full of peonies and lilies and all would be forgiven.

I saw an end to the piles of bills, the difficult teenagers, the vengeful ex-husbands, the disappointed parents.

I had no idea that cancer treatments were such a long, painful ordeal. I imagined the romantic tuberculosis in Anne of Green Gables. I thought I would waste away, becoming prettier and more fragile. And then perhaps, when my cheek and hipbones were sharp as Kate Moss or Bella Hadid's, I would disappear in a puff of smoke.

Instead, everything got worse. Like what Mick Jagger says about not always getting what you want. I got what I needed to change my point of view.

It was then that I started telling everyone I wasn't sick any more. I told my three daughters—who I call "The Amazons," because they were a seemingly tough pack of New York City schoolgirls—to pray, meditate, and focus on my being well by my oldest daughter's 17th birthday in early February.

I told my doctors that I wouldn't need any more chemotherapy. I wouldn't have surgery or radiation or anything else. I told the same to my friends and family. My doctors and chemo nurses at Memorial Sloan Kettering (who truly wanted me to live) said I was in denial. They sent psychiatrists who told me alternative cancer cures were "fairy stories." My oncologist yelled on the phone, "If you walk out of here now, you will kill yourself—you will be dead—in 12 weeks. Is that what you want to do to your children?"

I finally found an integrative oncologist called Mitchell Gaynor and I told him, "I am going to believe I am well. And if I believe I am well, I will be well."

He looked me straight in the eye and said, "Most spiritual traditions would agree with you. I believe you will be fine." I practically burst into tears at his confidence. He gave me a comprehensive list of supplements and told me to take my meditation more seriously.

Sadly, he was a member of the establishment, so he had to sell me upstream. A week later, his secretary called to say that my oncologist had contacted him. Dr. Gaynor wouldn't see me again unless I finished the course of chemotherapy and had surgery. Fear of malpractice suits, I guess. But the fact that he believed me, even for a few days, gave me the strength to keep going. Despite seeming cheerful and healthy, in September of 2015, Dr. Gaynor died of a supposed suicide.

I knew there was another way. There were a lot of other ways and I was determined to find them. Yes, you can even do surgery, chemotherapy, and radiation and combine what they call CAM (complementary alternative medicine) and diet and supplements and get even better results than the doctors thought possible. But you don't have to choose a single path. There are many.

What I discovered is that there are lots of other ways. Polarity therapy, Reiki, Brennan healing, Acupuncture, nutrition, exercise, prayer, meditation, hypnosis, psychic healing, homeopathic medicine, medicinal oils, herbal medicines, Chinese medicine, Ayurvedic medicine, Native American medicine—and that's just a tiny corner.

Every person with cancer needs to put together her own arsenal of healers. Cancer is so systemic that unless it's in its earliest stages, no single method alone will do it. You must take the time to put together the people who can support your journey. It doesn't require a lot of money, but it does require determination.

YOU CAN DO IT.

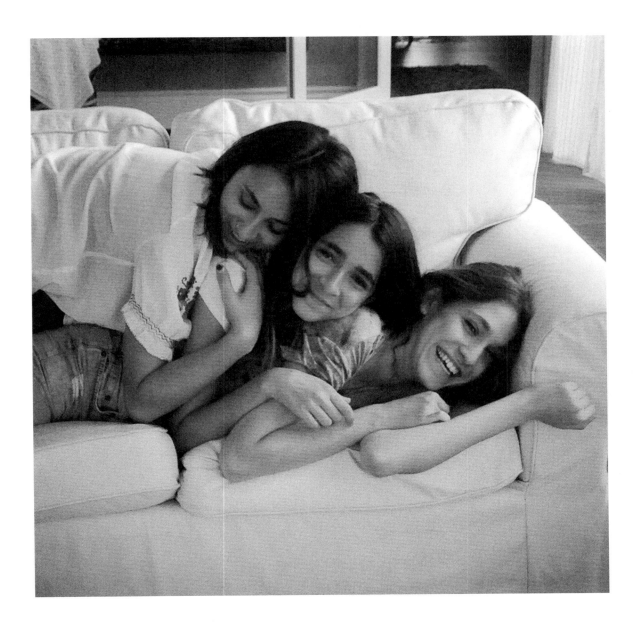

TABLE OF CONTENTS

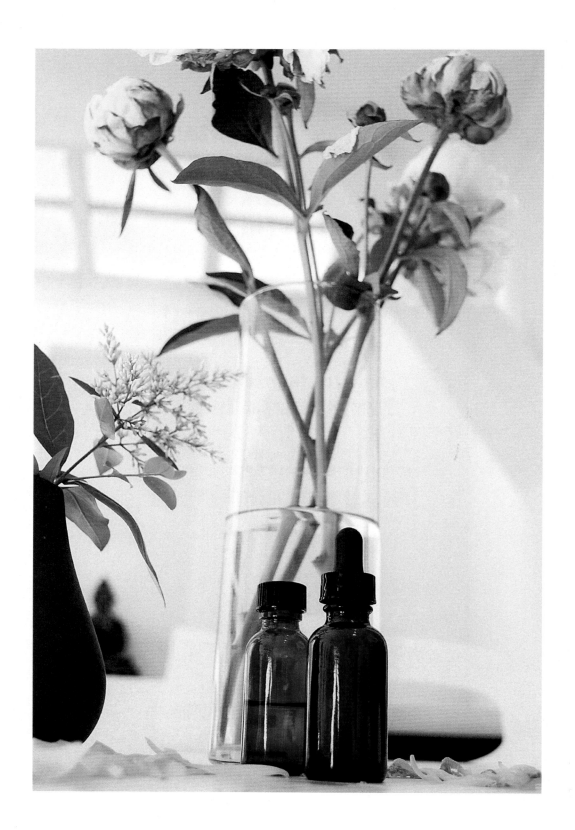

Be Here Now.
Facing the Diagnosis.

What you do when you hear the C-Word.

CHAPTER ONE: Be Here Now

When you get that phone call, or that email, or simply those words from your doctor's mouth, what will you do?

That is the reason for this book.

Everyone has those moments in their lives. Those moments which are so sharp and clear they become pivots for everything that happens next. Time freezes like a glitch, a vibrating frame in a downloaded movie.

You are suddenly aware of every detail around you. The sound of the clock humming, the smell of the floor cleaner and the rubbing alcohol, the hard chair underneath you. You remember the metallic taste in your mouth, the light, maybe it's late afternoon and it's just started to drizzle. Your heart is beating harder and it feels like your skin is humming. Even your own breath sounds deafening. Those moments where you realize that everything after this will be different. Quite often, you don't cry or move, because it's all you can do to choke out the words.

You want to ask, "Are you sure?" about 10 million more times because it all seems so unreal.

That's what it feels like when you have a life-shattering incident. Whether it's your dog getting hit by a car or a disaster in your house or losing a family member or someone telling you, "You have cancer."

That's why I am writing to you.

Do this first:

Breathe.

Breathe slowly and deeply. Let your lungs fill with air until it feels like you've expanded into the whole room. Exhale, exhale, exhale until every last bit of that air and even some that's been left inside the dark corners of your body is gone.

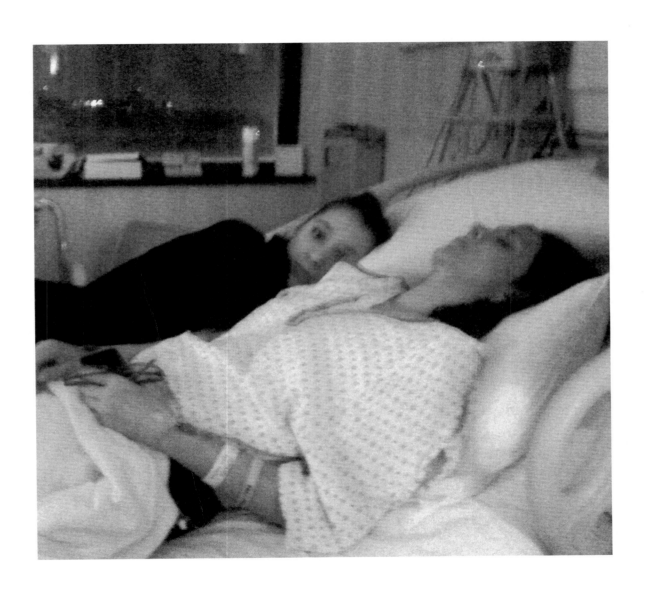

Do it again. As slowly as you can manage. Feel the air brushing your nostrils and lips as it comes and goes.

Cancer is not a death sentence.

I will repeat that over and over again. Cancer is not the end of the world. It is not a death sentence. Do not let the terror take you over. I am with you here.

If you're so scared you're about to die then the doctor—any doctor, good or bad—in a calm and authoritative voice, will tell you what to do. And like a robot, you will just listen and do what you are told.

And that can get you in a lot of trouble. Fear does that.

You won't be able to make the decisions that could change your quality of life.

Cancer is an intense, systemic illness, but chances are, it will not kill you. More and more people are contracting cancer but more and more are surviving cancer. The numbers are increasing every day. The number of ways in which people are taming their cancer are growing exponentially. When you are ready, check out the numbers on the National Cancer Institutes or even the American Cancer Society. Today, the chances cancer will kill you are less than 20%. If you saw those chances of rain on a Saturday, you might not change your picnic plans.

Many people who suffered through the worst kinds of cancer are not only surviving but thriving. Living better, happier, and more alive than ever before. If you think about it, you may discover that many people you know have experienced cancer on some level and recovered.

Depending on how far the cancer has progressed in your body, you will have to work harder to get past it. But if you are willing to put the work into it, it's more than likely that you will. That's what I want to help you do.

The diagnosis feels like the end of the game. It's the opposite. A major illness can shake you to the core and then force you to make the major changes your life needs to get to the next level.

You are intelligent, questioning, caring. Value yourself and the form G-d (Divine Intelligence, Yahweh, Hashem, Allah, Jesus, Brahma, the Great Spirit) gave you. There is a reason you are here. We need you here.

This book is full of lists to make remembering things easier. So here are most crucial pieces of information to know when you are diagnosed are these three things. When you hear the c-word, breathe and know that you don't have to be scared or give up. Know this:

1. After you drink a glass of water, *you don't have to do anything.* Not right now. Nothing

will happen tomorrow. Not even the next day. No matter what they tell you, you have a little time to process it.

The force of all the information you're being told and all the information you don't yet know is coming at you so fast that it feels like you're in a wind tunnel.

If you just surrender yourself to what you're told, you won't consult other doctors, you won't know if this is the best treatment for your body, you won't know if you like the facility you are in. You won't even know if you like the way your doctor speaks to you.

If, on the other hand, you take a breath and say, "I'll go home and put things in order and come in tomorrow morning," you will have a little time to remember that you are a capable and functioning adult. You will remember that you have options. You can say, "I don't want a transfusion, I want..."

You will remember that you walked in on your own and you can walk out.

2. Cancer doesn't mean you will die. Say that to yourself 10 or 50 or 200 times. Scream, sob, cry, yell at whoever you think can take it (though not your partner because he or she is terrified too, and not your kids, no matter how old they are). Even if your doctor or your tarot card reader says that you are going to die, it doesn't mean you will. Give yourself love and compassion. But keep telling yourself that.

3. Whatever you do, do not go through it alone. Remember that you are never, ever alone. Mobilize your friends and family. Mobilize your neighbors. If you don't have people close by, maybe mobilize people you've talked to on the street. Ask. People really want to help.

Shock and panic are normal reactions. That's what I felt like. Even though I knew it was coming, I had no idea how hard it would hit me. Discovering that you actually have cancer, not hypochondria, is really scary.

Breathe. Then go home.

When you get there, take your coat and shoes off.

Or do whatever you do to relax and feel safe. Keep breathing slowly, deeply. If you've ever done yoga or given birth to a child, you know how to breathe to slow down time. Maybe make a cup of tea. Do something ordinary and ritualistic. Lie or sit down in whatever part of your home is your sanctuary.

For me, I like to lie in my bed with a pillow over the top half of my head. The reason for the pillow is that I used to sleep under a dazzling skylight. Sometimes I don't want to be dazzled any more than I have been already.

That afternoon, I closed the door but I could still hear the muffled noises of the yapping dog and my daughters arguing in the kitchen. That made me feel calmer. Like life is going on as usual and everything will be all right. Though, I didn't really believe it would be all right. I lay in my bed and felt sorry for myself. I felt desolate and abandoned.

The thing is, the one journey in life we make totally alone is death. One way to make sure you stay alive and vital is to stay connected to the people you love and care about. It doesn't have to be a spouse, it doesn't even have to be a family member, if they are not available.

Statistics show that people who get sick—it doesn't matter what it is—are more likely to survive (and often come out healthier) if they have a social network. Real physical world friends, not just Facebook. That said, I had a huge network of family and friends online who read my posts and commented on my pictures and sent me words of encouragement and moral support. Facebook turned out to be a very useful tool for keeping family and friends in farflung places informed. A writer friend of mine, Robert Goolrick, put together beautiful Facebook pages for friends with cancer. They become Facebook "parties" with everyone posting "presents"—pictures, poems, stories, videos—for the recovering person. It's a way to get in contact with people when you really don't feel well enough to get dressed and come downstairs.

But it's not enough.

In the beginning, you need people who can show up. Real life people you can call and talk through what just happened. People who come over and listen to you rant about the craziness of it all. Even people who come over and talk about their own dramas because sometimes it's nice to be distracted. It gives you perspective.

And today, before it's all started, while you still have a bit of quiet—rest.

Then, when you feel a little better, call up a friend or family member. Start with one who isn't going to freak out or go into a panic or tell you it's not true. Someone who won't interrupt you 10 times while you are talking to ask you questions that you don't know the answers to and will make you more panicked. Usually, it's good to call someone whose strength is staying calm and listening in a crisis.

Talk it through so you can make sense of it in your mind.

Whatever you do, don't give into the frenzy that some doctors and acquaintances seem to want you to feel. You don't need surgery this second. Unless you are hemorrhaging to the point of losing consciousness, you don't need a blood transfusion in an hour. The good thing (if you feel like being Pollyanna about it) about cancer as opposed to trauma is that you don't need to make an immediate decision. It's not like getting hit by a car or falling out of a tree. You made it this far and you will probably get up tomorrow morning.

I found I just wanted someone to curl up in bed with me. Since I don't have a husband or a partner and I don't like the dog in my bed (I have white sheets!) I called my 9-year-old. Rara is the youngest so she is used to being babied and cuddled. Being held and touched apparently increases the strength of your immune responses, so it was probably the right thing to do.

When I went for my first visit to Memorial Sloan Kettering after I had been diagnosed, one of the two doctors who dropped everything to see me said, "You can't leave, I am checking you into the hospital right away."

My heart was beating so hard, all the blood rushed to my head, pumping behind my eyes and throbbing through my skull. It blocked out my vision and my hearing as my adrenaline will kicked in. I said, "I can't do that. I have three kids at home. I can't just go to a doctor's appointment and not come back." I felt like they had just kicked the floor out from under me.

In retrospect, I had a very aggressive, fast-moving cancer. At that point, it was probably stage 4. I was hemorrhaging so much so that I had very little blood left in my body. I was gray and skinny and exhausted. I said, "But my daughter has a ballet performance she's been working on for months, it's tomorrow. Can't I come tomorrow evening?"

Even in my case, it would have been fine to have waited a day. (Though probably smart to miss the ballet). Unless you are in the very last stages, cancer will NOT kill you overnight. (And if it did, wouldn't you rather be surrounded by people you love?)

So take a day or two. If you can get time off work, great. But if you can't, enjoy being distracted. Call a few more friends and see if they know about your kind of cancer. Remember that cancer acts differently in almost everyone. The first protocol is not always the most effective.

Once you start treatment, it's harder to seek out other options because the treatment can be so time-consuming, tiring, and overwhelming. There are a lot of different kinds of cures, not all in hospitals. Different cancers respond to different kinds of medicines— whether they are surgery, chemotherapy and/or radiation—or whether they are nutritional or energetic.

I believe it's crucial to combine several methods of recovery. Take the time to understand your particular cancer and how it works because once you get on the medical merry-go-round, they often don't have the time to explain it to you.

If you can't do it yourself, ask your friends to help you explore. Personally, I was so frightened that I couldn't do much research. The anxiety made reading impossible. I was too choked up to talk on the phone. I was ashamed and didn't believe anyone would have taken my calls.

Take some time to decide if you like the doctors. Check to see if you feel like they listen to you. If you go into treatment at their facility, you will see a lot of them. Ask your friends for recommendations

This is a good time to meditate. Let me clarify. Meditation means different things. Sometimes, it's sitting cross-legged on a cushion or a yoga mat. Other times, it's lying in bed. It could be a walk or sitting at your kitchen table looking out the window. What I mean is, take the time to reflect. Don't beat yourself up. Instead, take a little time alone to think and feel. Give yourself all the love and slack you can.

Even if you just have 15 minutes to sit in another room and make a decision—take that time and meditate and take your body's temperature—psychically. Take a look at your life and your lifestyle, you may notice the triggers that made you ill. Those kind of things jump out at you at crucial moments. You might have a moment of clarity.

Breathe slowly and try to imagine the energy in your body. Think about what feels ok and where you feel pain or energy blocks. Whatever happens, try and be aware of your being before the doctors start telling you what they think.

Always keep in mind, this is **YOUR** body. You know it. You own it. You've lived in it for years.

This is also good time to start drawing your roadmap. Think about how you want to tell your family and the people dependent on you. Think about how you might want to deal with it at work. Think about how you might want to deal with your treatments. Go over whatever the doctor told you. Just think and let ideas pop into your head. Ask your friends to report back with any research they've found. There is A LOT. 169,000 and counting books on cancer on Amazon.com. That doesn't even include videos, blogs, treatment centers, and quackery.

Whatever you do, don't worry too much, you're writing in pencil right now. Nothing is set in stone.

Let your mind wander, but try to keep it as calm as you can. Get into the flow. Maybe lie in bed or take a walk. Think about how to make the fewest waves in the river rushing around you. Or maybe it's time for you to make a lot of waves?

Let me add one more thought. This will liberate you as you make your decisions about your treatment.

Don't be afraid of death.

The reason is, when you're dead, you've got nothing to worry about.

Read some accounts of people who "died" and came back, if you don't believe me. Eben Alexander's Proof of Heaven is a good one.

No bills. No aches. No painful treatments. No creditors. No obnoxious relations (or teenaged children or ex-husbands or ex-wives).

No cancer.

What you should be scared of is having your quality of life affected. Be scared of getting a treatment that doesn't work for your body or your kind of cancer. Or a chemotherapy doses that is too strong for you. Or the after-effects of the drugs you are given. Be scared of having a doctor or caregiver who doesn't listen to your concerns or explain the details of your treatment in advance.

Be scared of not really living.

But don't give up on yourself because you're intimidated.

The power is in your hands.

When you feel a teensy bit calmer, you can tell your family.

I loved *The Big* C TV series. I understand both the power and liberation of holding on to a secret. Laura Linney, the main character, chose not to tell her family she had cancer. By not telling anyone, she was able to live without anyone's judgments or input. She set herself free. She (and the audience) always had the power of knowing what was REALLY happening.

I wish I could have done that. But I am horrible with secrets. I can barely keep the contents of Christmas presents quiet. I need to talk through things. I need to hear other people's ideas because they help me clarify mine.

Also, I didn't want my family members to hear it from anyone else first.

In my case, it was morning on a sunny Saturday. I'd gotten back in bed, pretending to read the newspaper in a shaft of brilliant light. I shouted for my kids to come upstairs. Often on the weekends, we all lolled around in bed and cuddled and read the paper and had our tea together. They came over, jumping and rolling on the bed and wrestling with each other like a pack of puppies. They were 15, 12, and 9. I said, "Hey, stop for a minute. I have something to tell you. You know I've been really sick and tired lately? I wanted you guys to know first. I have a rare kind of cancer."

Of course, that stopped everyone right away. They all froze. No better conversation killer. From what I remember, even the dog stopped yapping.

Then they asked the usual question that kids ask. "Are you going to die?"

I said, "Everyone is going to die some time. So yes, I am going to die. But I am not going to die tomorrow. Probably not for a while. And even when I do die, whenever that is, I am not going to disappear. I am going to be right there watching you. So don't think that if I die you get to act crazy and do what you want. I will be keeping an eye on you."

In retrospect, that's the best way to tell your kids. It was fatalistic and harsh. I didn't yet know what I know now. I believed what I saw in movies and TV shows. A character gets cancer because they are about to be taken off the air. It's a dramatic death and it absolves them of all of their past sins. I thought I was going to die. I thought it was better to be straightforward and realistic.

My now 21-year-old remembers that I told her, "I have been diagnosed with cancer and will die in three months." That's not how I recall it, but that doesn't matter. The point is, there's no reason to be too morbid and final, especially with your kids, no matter how seriously you want people to take it.

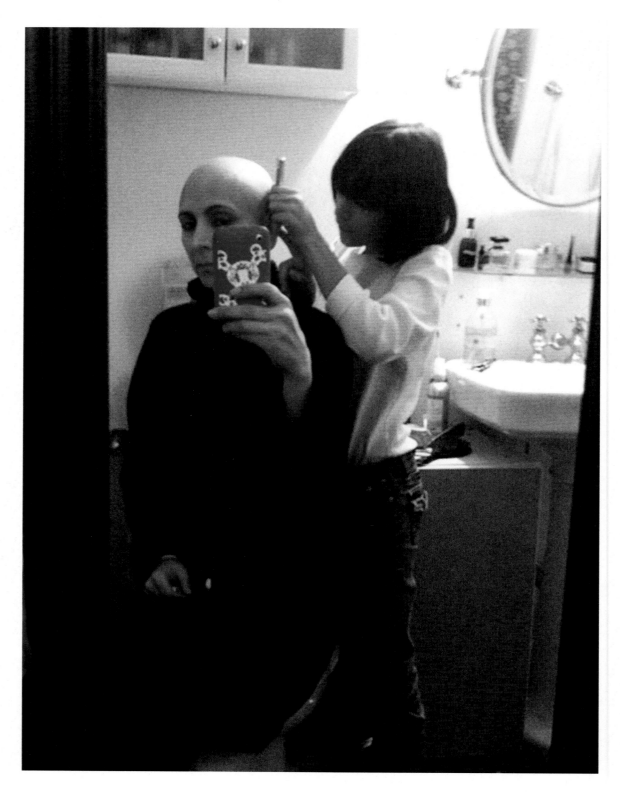

Fortunately, when they got my diagnosis—two or three weeks after my biopsy —my doctor's office hadn't been able to reach me so they called my brother. At least, I didn't have to inform him. To my parents who were in India then, I said, "I have a rare uterine cancer," I said, "I don't know all the details, but I will let you know when I do."

My brother, being the amazing autodidact that he is, started doing research right away. A writer friend, Zia Jaffrey, helped my brother and, before I even started treatment, I had an entire dietary plan mapped out for me. They took a lot of information from Cancer Tutor's cancer diet, which is based on the idea that "100% of everything you eat should be in the category of 'Foods that contain nutrients that kill the cancer cells, stop the spread of cancer, or in some other way help treat the cancer.'" In natural medicine, you cannot treat the cancer unless you treat the diet because everything you ingest is the terrain or basis for the treatment.

Thus, my fourth key piece of advice for someone who has just been diagnosed with cancer is this: The minute you find out, give up sugar. It is EVIL. By sugar, I mean anything that turns into sugar in your body — cane sugar, corn syrup, beet sugar, honey, maple syrup, agave, stevia, white flour, white rice, potatoes, fruit, some people even say ALL grains and even all carbohydrates except for vegetables. A doctor friend argued with me about this so here's some concrete evidence. German biologist Otto Heinrich Warburg won a Nobel Prize in 1931 for discovering that the metabolism of malignant tumors is dependent on glucose consumption. Insulin production triggers inflammation. People who eat low-sugar Asian diets tend to have five to 10 times fewer hormonally-driven cancers than those with diets high in sugar and refined foods. While you're doing that, you might also give up caffeine, eat organic (to avoid unnecessary pesticides), and give up animal products.

For the record, at my first and second ultrasounds—at two separate hospitals, St. Vincent's and Mount Sinai, just a week apart—they discovered a tumor that was four centimeters and growing rapidly. A few days after I was told I had cancer, I gave up sugar, wheat, dairy, and all animal products.

Two weeks' later, when I was admitted to Memorial Sloan Kettering, I had another ultrasound. The tumor was two centimeters. It had shrunk by half.

The doctor told me this may have been the different ultrasound machines, but the speed at which my cancer responded to the chemotherapy had the nurses shouting, "Oh my God, it's a miracle!"

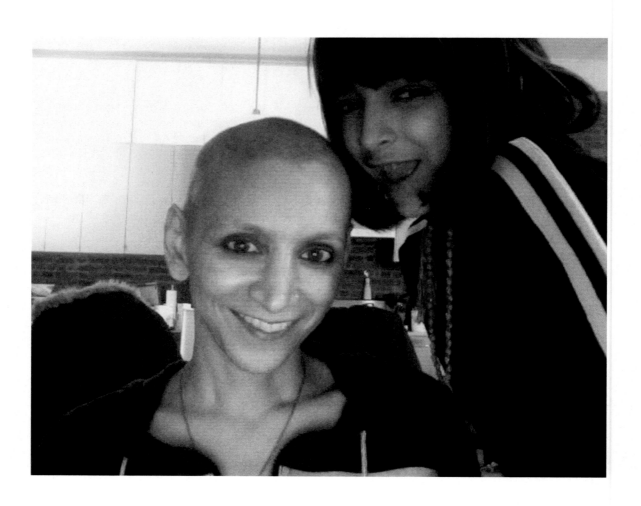

Start Here. Ten Easy Things You Can Do Right Now.

(to get your cancer under control)

CHAPTER TWO: Start Here, or Ten Things You Can Do Right NOW to Change Your Outcome.

One day, as a Scottish chemo nurse was sticking an IV into my arm (still feel nauseated just thinking about it), she murmured to me, "It does seem that people often develop cancer after an emotional crisis."

In my case, I can almost pinpoint when it happened. It was the beginning of March 2009. I always feel optimistic in the spring. The light changes and there's the smell of the thawing earth. In the old apartment, we woke to sun streaming in and the sound of birds in the park.

In the fall of 2008, my freelance career suddenly ran dry and by the spring, my savings and perfect credit rating were decimated. We were on the verge of being evicted from our apartment in the building we'd lived in for 17 years.

I had one goal: to keep my kids fed, clothed, and in one place until the end of the school year, especially because it was a crucial high school year for my oldest.

My now very successful exhusbands combined forces to respond to my request for regular child support based on their incomes. They sent me a combined email: "We are unwilling to support your unsustainable lifestyle..." one suggested I go on food stamps. They told me to fire the housekeeper/babysitter and have the kids look after each other. I cried and begged them to at least intervene on our behalf with the landlord. If they couldn't do that, perhaps they could help cover some of the costs of adding a bathroom and some kitchen cabinets in the old storefront I was turning into a family apartment. Needless to say, my requests went unheeded. Many mornings, I scrambled to find healthy food for the girls' breakfasts.

We downscaled, sold our clothes and furniture, moved into a tiny basement apartment around the corner using shopping carts, outgrown strollers, and helpful students. I made the place habitable myself with endless trips to IKEA, maxing out my credit cards. My landlord sued me. My other exhusband used this opportunity to sue me for all the money I asked for that he didn't give us. They set up an emotional lynching and left all of us reeling.

26

I fell behind on the mortgage payments.

The place started flooding every time it rained. I used the tiny amounts of credit on my cards to turn the electricity and the cable back on when it would get turned off. I complained to the building management and they ignored me. The wiring on my car was eaten by rats. (What's amazing is that the new owners found out that all that water damage had actually decayed the beams holding up my floor! It's a wonder we didn't crash straight down to the basement! I am grateful for that.)

I'm laughing as I type this because I sound like Job in the Bible and I was not as sanguine as he was.

(Recently, a friend of mine got mad at me for swimming every day because chlorine increases cancer risks, some say by 93%)

Here's the thing I believe: Cancer is caused by stress and sadness.

Stress, tension, anxiety, grief, anger—whatever combination of all of those things—as long as they are unresolved.

You know when you tell a friend not to do something unhealthy and he or she says, "My grandmother smoked a pack a day and lived on lard and whiskey until she was a healthy 107..."?

The reason, apart from sturdier genetics and the changing chemical landscape, that some people don't get sick is because you can be exposed to all kinds of horrid things and nothing can get to you until your emotional state lets your body down. It's a way of checking out.

I have a one friend who never smoked a day in his life and got lung cancer, serious enough for surgery. I had a young friend who got cancer in his spine and was gone before he was 27. He'd had a very painful childhood and was a very angry person.

I'm not saying that these people consciously wished to die. But sometimes, the pressure is just too much.

So I started chemotherapy and discovered that dying of cancer was not nearly as romantic as consumption. Instead, it was painfully slow and awful, no matter how aggressive your cancer was. I also saw how hard watching me fall apart was on my daughters. That's when I decided I was going to get well. And fast.

I was lucky on one side. My particular cancer had a 70% success with chemotherapy (30% death rate is still high, isn't it?). When I was diagnosed, I had black lesions in my brain and lungs according to the scans. Did it recede, or was it misdiagnosed? Apparently, that's how oncologists often explain the inexplicable, according to David Servin-Schreiber's Anti-Cancer: A New Way of Life. I put it down to giving up sugar, caffeine, and animal products as soon as I got the phone message from my Gynecologist and—as I said—the tumor shrank by half two weeks after I changed my diet.

So I told my oncologist that I was well.

She said, "You're in denial."

I said, "Cancer is the most psychosomatic disease there is. So I am going to believe that I am well and then I will be well."

She said, "We don't subscribe to that sort of thing at Memorial Sloan Kettering. We don't believe cancer is some sort of punishment or there's some reason. We believe cancer just happens."

I smiled, "I don't think it's a punishment either. But I also don't think it's random."

In some ways, cancer can feel like a reward. A get-out-of-jail-free card. Like In Mark Twain's *Huckleberry Finn*, Tom Sawyer and Huck get to go their own funerals and hear everyone saying nice, regretful things about them. People are so scared of cancer. It seems so incredibly bad, that they almost HAVE to feel sorry. You get to experience the I'll-bet-they'll-be-sorry-now in real life.

When you're emaciated and bald with bloodshot eyes, most people feel uncomfortable being mean to you (however, often the people you hope to spite manage to go right ahead—and then other people just run away from you).

Thus, the cutting-off-your-nose-to-spite-your-face pleasure is pretty short-lived.

Eventually, even nice people get tired of being nice to you.

So here's the second thing I believe:

There is a cure for cancer.

Actually, curing cancer is sort of like curing a cold. I don't mean to make too light of it, because a cold can turn into pneumonia or bronchitis and then it's a lot harder to cure, and sometimes, there's a part of you that just gets tired and gives up.

Like colds or viruses, there is only so much the medical professionals can do. If you want to get well, you have to commit to it yourself. You have to drink the soup and take the vitamin C and get rest and put yourself first for a little while. And you have to be willing to trade all those people being nice to you for a big fight, both with yourself and your friends and family and doctors. You have to own it yourself. It is not easy.

But if you want to stay around for little while longer, it is worth it.

This is my first advice if you even suspect the c-word (or any other chronic or systemic illness). This is what you do for yourself while all the doctors and relatives are running around you trying to figure out what's wrong and how to pinpoint and treat it. I am not a doctor so I am not trained to suggest medical treatments, but I promise that taking these actions will make you feel better.

START HERE

1. Stop eating simple sugars (including fruit, honey, potatoes, white flour), anything that causes inflammation or possible allergies, (including peanuts, soy, corn, dairy, shellfish), caffeine, and ALL animal products.

Every chance you get, eat organic. If you can be choosy, eat cruciferous vegetables like they are going out of fashion. Kale, swiss chard, watercress, broccoli, cabbage, brussel sprouts, cauliflower. You will just have to live with the gas. Some people find that adding lots of ginger to one's diet helps with that. (There are recipes in **Chapter Ten**).

Even better, juice that kale and swiss chard and mustard greens, too. If you can get yourself a juicer and you have someone to work it, or you can afford to buy freshly-made organic juice outside, drink 16 to 20 oz of green juice at least once a day. Drink even more if you can. If you can get it cold-pressed, fabulous.

You can also eat them as sprouts!

When you juice, skip the fruit. Fruit is good for you, but right now you can't take the sugar and even if it's organic, it can be questionable.

2. Start drinking water chlorine filtered out, if you can) like crazy. But don't drink water from plastic bottles if you can avoid it.

Tension dehydrates you. It also spikes your blood pressure. The best way to lower your blood pressure and soothe your body is to increase your fluids.

At the very least, try to drink three liters a day to flush all the junk (and what the cruciferous vegetables might be killing) out of your system. If you can, or some natural/ organic baking soda to your water. In natural medicine, the idea is that the more alkaline your system, the more your own immune system can kick in and fight the aggressors.

3. Rest. Rest. Rest. It's like a cold, remember? Give your body a break so it can fight it. Exercise is good for preventing cancer but when you're in an outbreak—just like the flu—you need to rest up. If you're a mom, this is a chance to skip the ballet recitals and teacher conferences. Do not drag yourself around. Listen to your body. Turn off your phone. Close the door. Don't fight with your husband(s)—ex and present. Tell your kids to be nicer.

4. Get some heat. One little known fact about cancer is that it lowers your body temperature. You feel cold all the time. It's sort of like the way you get cold after eating a really big meal. All your blood rushes to your stomach to help it digest and the rest of you gets no love.

When you have cancer, all your blood seems to rush to the area of the cancer and heat it up and the rest of you gets cold. What seems to work is hypothermia. If you have no access to a sauna, get a bio-mat. They are expensive (around $700 for a small one and $1700 for a large). There are a lot of places to buy them, but they last for five or six years and lying on one really makes you feel better. The idea is to lie on it (three times a day) for 40 minutes on its highest setting and get all sweaty. This makes your body think you have a fever and it supercharges your immune system to fight back. Here's what the National Cancer Institute has to say about hypothermia: "Hyperthermia (also called thermal therapy or thermotherapy) is a type of cancer treatment in which body tissue is exposed to high temperatures. Research has shown that high temperatures can damage and kill cancer cells, usually with minimal injury to normal tissues. Many studies have shown a significant reduction in tumor size when hyperthermia is combined with other treatments." A Japanese doctor, Dr. Nakamachi Nobuhiro Yoshimizu, found he had good results using the bio-mat for 40-60 minutes at a time, three times a day for eight weeks at a time—shrinking and dissolving tumors. The heat on the cancer cells made them more susceptible to the cancer killing protocol. His book is called *The Fourth Treatment for Medical Refugees* and shows the results of the bio-mat use on a number of different cancers.

If you do decide to get chemo, the mat is a good way to recover when you come home wrecked at the end of a session. It also might make your chemo more effective.

Personally, I found the bio-mat most useful when I had to give myself injections to make my bones produce more blood cells. This gave me incredible pains in my hips and lower back. The only thing that relieved the pain was lying on the mat.

5. Breathe. Try pranayama breathing. Prana means life force in Sanskrit and this kind of breathing is an Ayurvedic and Yogic technique with proven health benefits. Breathe slowly and expansively, be generous with your body. Breathe in through your nose. Fill your ribcage, fill your stomach with your breath. Then release it slowly. Try and make each inhale as long as each exhale. Enjoy it. The oxygen will help alkalize your body and strengthen your immune system. It will help the platelets in your blood swim freely.

Maybe try alternate nostril breathing. It's good for helping the left and right side of your brain and body be more connected.

Any time a new wave of fear or anxiety hits you, give yourself a few minutes of sitting still focusing on your breathing and the sensations in your body. Be present to the things in your body that are working well.

Slowly imagine a light moving from the top of your skull down through the inside your body, illuminating it with sparkling light. Imagine it dissolving all blocks and worries, especially in your solar plexus. Every time you feel frightened again, breathe. Slowly.

6. Get some energy. I highly recommend a powerful supplement called Polymva

It's a combination of palladium, alpha lipoic acid and B-vitamins that is both bio-available and crosses the brain-blood barrier. I explain how it works in **Chapter Eight**. In my case, it made the chemo hyper-effective and radically improved my quality of life (QOL).

While I didn't use it, I've seen people have great results with something called Essiac tea. This Native American herbal formula soothes your digestive tract, reduces inflammation, inhibits tumor growth, and detoxes and nourishes your body. I drink it these days as a prophylactic. (More in **Chapter Nine**).

I've also seen people shrink away tumors using medicinal oils like frankincense and myrrh (there's a reason the three kings brought them as gifts). I now know three people who massaged these oils on to their tumors and had them melt away. I don't know the exact dosage but they are worth exploring. Marijuana in the form of cannabinoid or CBD oil has been shown to have incredible anti-tumor properties, both ingested and applied topically, but since it was not legally available in New York City at that time, I never tried it.

The combination of PolyMVA and people praying for me and over me before every session had my doctors running into my room saying, "It's a miracle!" after every new blood test result came in.

Again, I have no formal medical training or authority, but this is what worked for me.

Think about supplementing your own spiritual energy reserves with energy healing. I went to a healer called Penney Leyshon who gave me clarity and helped me gather my strength and resist the paralyzing fear and confusion. Again, the idea is to truly believe and know you are well.

Some people find other kinds of energy work—hypnosis, Polarity, Brennan, or Reiki—give them clarity and serenity. I recommend you experiment with everything until you find what works for you. Recently, scientists have done studies showing the effectiveness of energy healing in resolving cancers.

There have recently been a series of studies that show that energy work actually shrinks tumors.

7. Slow down. Think it through. If you can do the other stuff—especially the first two —remember that you DO have time. Really.

There are health issues that require immediate and urgent medical attention, like when you've been in a serious accident, or had a stroke or a heart attack, you are bleeding, or have a broken bone. But for the most part, with cancer (and lots of other illnesses), if you are well enough to be out walking around, you have time to do some research and understand your options.

Don't rush into anything.

Take a deep breath. If you can't think straight, ask your friends to help you. Right at the beginning, lots of people will have the energy to help. Use them while you can, because they will burn out.

8. Know that you're scared. So is your doctor. And so are all of your family members and your friends. That's why they try and rush you into instant steps to deal with the cancer. Cancer is one of those weird diseases that no one understands. It behaves differently in almost every body it enters. Also, different cancers behave differently, so no one can give you a one-size-fits-all answer.

In my opinion, fear is best handled with faith. Every faith tradition will tell you the same thing. It doesn't matter which one you choose, just put your faith in a higher power. Choose the form that speaks to your heart.

My suggestion would be, after you get your diagnosis, to avoid your doctors and immediate family members because they will be acting out of panic.

Instead, find a close friend who has a bit of time and can give you some help from a distance. Better still, find a couple of (calm, practical, respectful) friends who can help you do research into your kind of cancer.

When I was diagnosed, I was so scared, I couldn't do much research because my anxiety made it impossible for me to understand what I was reading. I was exhausted from losing so much blood and the words jumped around the screen or the page and my thoughts all jumbled together.

I just wanted someone to tell me what to do.

But, like everything else in the world, when you stop making decisions for yourself, other people make them for you.

Own your cure.

9. Look after your soul. Remember that this is YOUR body and YOUR life. While you are resting and/or lying on your bio-mat, think about what you really want. Sometimes, checking out is the right thing. Sometimes, chemotherapy and surgery are what you feel most comfortable with. But remember that everything has risks and many have long-term side effects. In my case, my 14 weeks' of chemotherapy caused early menopause, osteoporosis, irreversible heart and kidney damage. Think about the kind of life you want afterwards.

Maybe you want to reduce your participation and let others help more. Maybe you want to play even harder.

Remember the story of *Rumplestiltskin?* The young maiden was willing to promise away her first-born son because she was in a panic—and she couldn't imagine that she would ever have that life. Are you trading your future for what might be a temporary stay?

PRAY, MEDITATE, VISUALIZE.

Oh also—whatever you do, **DON'T FEEL SORRY FOR YOURSELF.**

I mean, everyone has their moments where they stamp around the house and say, "It's just not fair! Why does this happen to ME?"

Or sob into their pillows and say, "Oh my God, Rachel married a great guy and has gorgeous kids and her marriage is perfect and they have such a nice house and why am I in this situation?"

But after that, get over it and put your problems in perspective. The nature of the world is that there is always someone who has things much worse than you (or I) do. Especially if you are middle class and living in the first world.

If you blame other people for your situation or feel like a victim, then you're in someone or something else's control—and how can you possibly get well?

Actually, this piece of advice works for just about everything. So get up, get going and laugh at the absurdity. You got yourself into this situation and you will get yourself out. If you really, really want to, you will.

10. Laugh. Watch idiotic funny movies. Ask people to tell you jokes. If you're a mum, tell your kids to come and cuddle up with you in bed and ask you riddles. Laughing is known to ramp up your immune system, too. The more you can laugh, the better. Stay away from people who make you sad or worried. It might seem hard but remember, you are saving your life here.

10 and a half. Keep the germs away. Wash your hands every time you're near a sink.

The Detox.
Learning How to Say No.

(to what you don't want.
Setting boundaries.)

CHAPTER THREE: How to Say No. The Detox.

Detox is a trendy word these days. It's thrown around, along with juice and water fasts and the master cleanse. It can include things like colonics, skin brushing, and hot mineral baths. It varies greatly depending on which doctor or theory you follow. It can also mean an emotional clearing. But you must be careful with detoxes because you are already physically weak and you don't want to take away too much.

Most alternative health books start with the detox. Before you can start healing, you need to get your body stronger and give it the support it needs to come back into balance.

I'm going to start with a relatively easy detox that you can probably do no matter how debilitated you are. And, it won't interfere with your chemotherapy or radiation if you choose to do them at the same time.

This is step two.

If you followed the first set of instructions, you don't have too far to go.

No Processed Foods, No Sugar, No Dairy, No Wheat, No Soy, Lots of Vegetables and Water.

You've already given up sugar, processed foods, non-organic foods, inflammatory foods like wheat and dairy, you're drinking three liters of water a day and you are eating a diet of 70-80% green vegetables—mostly cruciferous ones. Cruciferous vegetables contain sulphorafane, a cancer-fighting phytonutrient that helps stop the growth of cancer cells.

If you can't take so much roughage, I'd suggest starting slowly. Juice the veggies—try to drink at least 16 to 24 ounces of juice a day (you can subtract that from your three liters of water)—but don't add too much fruit! Fruit is too sugary. It both feeds your cancer and sabotages your health. Also, it's very hard to find pesticide-free fruit these days. If the juice is too intense, add more cucumber and/or lemon to cut the bitterness. If you feel like you really need some sweetness, add some organic green apple, carrots, or even pineapple, but not too much. If you are exhausted, ask a friend to help you juice.

Though it's best to drink the juice when it's fresh, you can even juice every other day. You can get friends to help on alternate days. If you live in a major metropolitan area in the

35

U.S., there may be juice bars where you can buy fresh cold-pressed juice. I suggest two caveats:

1. Keep an eye on how much fruit they put in and

2. Be careful that the juice has not been pasteurized or hpp processed because those two methods kill some of the enzymes, pre and probiotics that you need to strengthen your immune system and fight the cancer. For all the money you have to spend on the organic vegetable juice, you don't want something that has been sitting around in a plastic bottle for a month, you want every living bit of it!

Juicing deserves a book of its own because there are so many illness-kicking people having great success with it these days. Kris Carr of *Crazy Sexy Cancer* - find her inspiring work if you haven't seen it yet – has a book of recipes called *Crazy Sexy Juice*. Joe Cross of *Fat, Sick and Nearly Dead*, a documentary about how juicing saved his life, has a program called, Reboot with Joe, that also has lots of advice.

Another great way to bump up the cruciferous vegetables is by eating broccoli and kale sprouts. Three-day-old sprouts have 20 to 50 times the sulphorafane of regular broccoli or kale, according to a Johns Hopkins pharmacologist called Paul Talalay. If you buy your own organic seeds and use fresh water, you just need a tray—no garden—they are so easy a toddler could grow them and probably would enjoy the process.

Fix Your Teeth

In **Chapter Twelve**, I talk about a book by Ty Bollinger called *The 31-Day Home Cancer Cure*. He suggests your cure start with a trip to a holistic dentist. In 1951, a doctor called Josef Issels opened a holistic cancer center in Germany. It set a standard in beginning cancer treatment with the teeth. Issel's holistic cancer center still has a great deal of success.

Another way to deal with dental infections is oil-pulling—swooshing oil around your mouth for two to 20 minutes to neutralize bacteria and remineralize teeth. I do that every morning, using a half-a-tablespoon of raw coconut oil (instead of the traditional Ayurvedic sesame oil). Sometimes, I add in a drop of myrrh oil and 10 drops of golden seal extract to help clear any infections in my sinuses as well.

That is your basic physical detox. No matter what anyone says, I suggest you try it. More and deeper physical detoxes later. Now for the emotional detox.

Say No

I am always asked this question.

When faced with the enormous weight of the medical establishment and the cancer industry, along with the battalions of family members and friends who told me I was a selfish, unrealistic, irresponsible mother with a death wish, how did I say no?

How do you make a decision based on the quiet voice of your intuition when you're scared out of your skin? And when almost every person of repute is telling you that your intuition might be deadly wrong.

How do you do what you feel in your gut is right for you and your body?

This is critical.

Toddlers say "no" often and with conviction. "No green beans!" "No shoes!" It's simple.

Teenagers do it by rolling over and going back to sleep or ignoring their parents' text messages. It's all about creating a separate identity and learning to make your own boundaries. It's a crucial developmental step.

Eventually, though, as we grow up, we all learn the value of saying "yes," or at least, "oh, all right," most of the time. It's a necessary part of living in society. We get to work when we are told to be there, we do the laundry for the whole family, make dinner when we're exhausted.

The problem is that we—especially women—often forget that we need to assert our independence sometimes. Not just for the brief rush of power (and ensuing guilt) of doing what we want, but as a sort of self-protection. There is only so much you can do and if you don't learn to protect yourself, the world will eat you up.

I am not suggesting that the world is malicious, just that the people who love you most, who care most about you, sometimes don't realize that you are a human yourself who also has a responsibility to her/himself. That sometimes you need to tell them "no."

When you are sick, this can get even harder.

If you feel like your illness might respond better to a certain diet, let's say your own version of Alejandro Junger's Clean, Fred Bisci's Spartan diet, Norman Walker's juicing or Gerson therapy or any of the variations and options out there, you need to protect yourself from the people who love you and may have stayed up all night baking your favorite brownies or frying samosas.

If you are weak and tired (and don't even like brussel sprouts or broccoli, but somehow know that's what you need); you need to say, "No, thank you," to the person who brought cupcakes and the doctor who says, "What you eat doesn't really matter anyway."

For the hospital, here is your first bit of ammunition. In the land of the invalids, the squeaky wheel gets gets the oil. Statistically, patients who complain and demand attention get better care—and recover faster. The more active you are in the process, the better your care will be—mainly because you've lived in your body and you know it better than any doctor ever could.

I'm not suggesting you be nasty and mean to anyone—and especially not to the nurses because they really work hard—but that you stick to what you believe. Even doctors and nurses, when they stop to think, believe this.

The uncomplaining patient who quietly does what she or he's told tends to be forgotten in the rush. If you have unpleasant symptoms or side-effects and you don't demand that your doctor address them in some way, you run the risk of hurting yourself in the long run. The human body reacts differently to different drugs as well as different illnesses. It's possible that something that seems unimportant may turn out to be something serious.

That's why I suggest you listen to yourself and your body. Trust your intuition.

When you are sick, vulnerable, frightened, or even just intimidated, that is the time to say "no" and take your power back.

No, I don't want cortisteroids.

No, I don't want a medical student to give me spinal tap, I'd rather have someone with years of experience.

No, I can't walk there, I want a wheelchair.

No, I don't want a wheelchair, I'd rather walk myself. And please don't hold my arm, I'm not decrepit.

Even if every single person tells you that acupuncture or prayer or avoiding surgery or chemotherapy or radiation is a stupid thing to do, if you feel like something is not working for you, if you get a sinking feeling as you start do it, say "no." (Interestingly, my daughters never question my convictions.) You can change your mind at any time, don't let anyone tell you otherwise.

Nothing is set in stone. You ALWAYS have a choice.

Remember that. There is a patient's bill of rights that allows you to refuse any treatment that you don't feel is benefitting you. It means that your doctors need to explain what they are doing and why. Just because something has "always been done that way" or because something is the "standard protocol" doesn't mean it always works or it can't be improved upon.

In my case, I knew too many people who had suffered from the side-effects of chemotherapy and radiation. The cancer was defeated, but with many of my friends, it came roaring back in four or five years because the person's natural immune system was so decimated by the chemo. I've known people who were killed by the side effects of chemotherapy and radiation but I never met anyone who was killed by natural medicine. (That doesn't mean it doesn't happen or that natural medicine always works, but there are fewer side effects.)

While I am a big proponent of natural healing methods, there is a lot to be said for your state of mind. If you really have faith in whatever method you are using to get well, it is likely to work. If you have doubts, don't do it.

For me, I tried psychic healers, massage and craniosacral therapists, acupuncturists, integrative oncologists, Reiki healers, Brennan method healers, yoga teachers, nutritionists, and hypnotists. I chose them based on positive recommendations from others. If something felt good—and I found research supporting it—I kept doing it. If it didn't feel like it was doing me good or I didn't respond to the energy of the person, I stopped.

I really worked on not being intimidated by either the New Age machinery or the medical industry.

Cancer and other life-threatening ailments are big business. Too many people are scared or intimidated into spending a lot of money on treatments that don't work for them. Say "no."

Not to be too trite but in Legally Blonde Two, Elle Woods (Reese Witherspoon) uses a disappointing hair color as a metaphor.

She stands on a platform and says that if you "witness injustice" even to yourself, you need to use your voice. In other words, "Speak UP!" for what you need.

Sometimes you realize that part of the reason you got sick was that you didn't learn how to say "no" enough. No, I can't drive you there. No, I can't keep the kids this weekend so you and your girlfriend can go to a bed and breakfast. No, I can't cover that bill. No, you can't come have your lunch at my house just because you're in the neighborhood.

Years ago, my mother taught me the beginnings of saying no to authorities. "Well, the recipe calls for three cans of chicken broth, but I made some chicken stock myself so I will use that." Or "The doctor told me to take this, but it's making me feel sick, so I'm going to throw the pills away and call him."

Start small. But work on it.

It's not always nice to say no to the people who care about you. But it's better to be nice to yourself sometimes.

When I finally told my oncologist I would not do any more chemotherapy despite her recommendations, she said, "You'll be dead in 12 weeks."

When I told the psychiatrists who were sent to counsel me that there were other ways to cure cancer, they laughed and said, "Those are fairy stories."

That was almost eight years ago. (That doesn't mean I might not have a relapse anyway, but in the meantime, I've enjoyed my life at full speed and on my own terms.)

Be brave.

Say "no."

It could save your life.

What to Expect When You are Hospitalized.

How to shrink the hospital to fit you.

CHAPTER FOUR: When/If You Are Hospitalized

When When I was diagnosed with cancer, I walked into Memorial Sloan Kettering and the very beautiful and lovely (I swear, she is a ringer for Julia Roberts) surgeon said to me, "I can offer you a hysterectomy on Monday." This was Thursday evening. She spoke as if she were offering me a slice of cake. This brilliant young surgeon was famous for her robotic, laser optic surgery which was promised to have a faster recovery and smaller scars. She is devoted and talented woman.

I said, "I don't WANT a hysterectomy!" Given my gynecological surgeon's polite and pleasant tone, my response was rude, but honestly, she scared the hell out of me. And I was scared already because I'd been hemorrhaging for the past two months and it was exhausting just to walk a city block.

Fear does strange things to you.

When you've just been diagnosed with something horrid and possibly life threatening, you do what seems to be the rational thing, you go to the place where everything seems the most calm and organized, where everyone seems to have everything under control. The advertising for Cancer hospitals, especially places like Memorial Sloan Kettering which is known for its pervasive and convincing campaign, can make them seem like the best choice.

This seems smart. As consumers, when we really freak out, we go to the brand that is synonymous with the product. Kleenex for tissues. For luxury, Chanel or Hermes. Sony for televisions. In our house, it's the Apple store for anything computer-related.

However, as it turns out, those big huge predictable organizations and corporations are not always the best as we are all learning. You remember the old ways—if you feel queasy, drink syrup of coke or Canada Dry Ginger Ale (which does not have real ginger in it and the sugar combined with the carbonation will eat through your teeth and bones and give you kidney stones)—or if you have a headache, take Bayer or Advil (which can have a rebound effect and can harm your kidneys). Johnson's baby Shampoo is the safest, gentlest cleanser – but it's not. There is no longer safety in what seems to be "tried-and-true."

So back to the advice I keep repeating. No matter what your doctor tells you, listen respectfully (and have a friend with you, writing it all down so you can research the information) and then, make your own decision.

When you are thinking about care, think SMALL.

For example: McDonald's, which successfully feeds millions of people every day, has expertise in preparing food. However, its true area of expertise is quantity, consistency, making low-quality food taste good and in keeping profits high

Now compare McDonald's to your mum, who has learned how to make nutritious meals for four or five people every night for 30 to 40 years. In her case, the area of food expertise will be about care, higher quality ingredients, and taste. You can't always count on the consistency, but it is outweighed by the hands-on mindfulness of someone who loves you.

In other words, in my experience, for real care, the idea is to think small and personal.

Unless you are a wealthy, high-profile person, you will not get special attention at a factory. Even one that operates with precision. And, in many instances, even if you have special access, doctors are taught to look after you the way one is taught to bake. It's a formula. You follow certain actions in a particular order—like a recipe—and, assuming you followed the instructions correctly, you get certain reactions—like a golden brown cake.

In my mind, there are issues with the way some doctors practice, especially in areas that are systemic (as opposed to a cut that needs stitches or a broken bone that needs to be re-set). I don't blame the doctors as insurance companies limit the amount of time they can spend with each patient as well as an entire industry limiting their ability to think outside of the box.

1. The formula or protocol is generally one-size-fits-all and human beings are not. In the same way that our metabolism, blood pressure, weight, and muscle mass differ, even in families, our bodies heal differently and absorb and activate medications differently and feel pain differently. Doctors have a degree of leeway to experiment, but not much.

2. I wasat a party some months ago. I found myself talking to a young doctor who worked for an HMO where he ended up treating a lot of Latin American patients. He said, "What people are talking about more and more are the differences in ethnicities and how they needed to be treated." You already know that your ethnicity affects your hair and skin color and texture. Obviously, it affects how your cells and internal organs operate as well.

3. The formula only treats one piece of a problem. So you can bake a perfect cake, but what about the frosting and the decoration and the rest of the party? The fact is our bodies are all connected, so what happens in your liver can affect your skin. It's one of those things that they used to believe in ancient times. For instance, women had their left nostril pierced originally because it was meant to make childbirth less painful. Sadly, I can't tell you if it works because I didn't pay attention when my nose was being pierced and got it on the right nostril instead. I am still wondering why the piercing woman didn't ask why I wanted the wrong side until after the job was done.

42

Now, let's say it's a day or two or a week later and you've done your research and you've decided you like and trust the doctor and you're checking into the hospital.

Or let's say it's whenever the doctor tells you to come and your heart is in your throat and the research makes you even more scared and overwhelmed.

What you want to do is ask a friend to keep doing research on the protocol you are having to see if there are reasons to customize it for your body. Maybe a smaller dose can be just as effective.

And...

the hospital is a big place. You want to make it feel small and you want to feel loved.

You can do that. Just a little harder when you really feel horrid. But it all pays off. It's all about loving them back.

HOW TO SHRINK YOUR HOSPITAL

Let me prepare you. This is such a long series of directions that I have cut it up into three parts. However, I suggest you print it out and take it with you to make a checklist before you go to hospital. Or print it out for your friends or family members who have to go.

Here is the basic stuff I've learned through years of experience as a successful patient. If you read this and you know someone else who is unwell (not just cancer, because I also had shingles, meningitis, a rare liver virus, a spina bifida baby, and a ruptured ovarian cyst), please pass it on. Not everything is useful for everyone but some of it will definitely make a difference.

The idea is to turn your big, scary hospital into a small, loving place. You want to make it a place where they will really look after you. You can even cheer up everyone else along the way.

Here's a list of ways to do it, starting with the intangibles—which make the most difference.

PART ONE:

Your MOOD:

One of my best friends, Sancha Mandy, a beautiful writer herself, who has been in the hospital way too many times says this, "Be an optimistic fatalist." You know you have to do it. Be brave and walk in. Keep in mind that it will all go well. Speak to your angels and the Divine Source and ask them to keep you safe and protect you from the treatments as well as the illness.

Be appreciative and be kind to all the people who help you there. There are orderlies and administrators and cleaning people. It is a hard job looking after sick people, it's emotionally draining. If you're in a cancer hospital, it can be devastating. Imagine how hard it is to come in to work every day.

Pretend that you are actually a celebrity incognito or a princess (not the Lindsay Lohan kind of celebrity. Think Audrey Hepburn in *Roman Holiday*). Be elegant, generous and kind. Behave with the grace of a princess and people will treat you like one.

Thank people.

Your NURSES

Make friends with all of your nurses. Learn their names if you can. Ask them how they are. You'd be surprised how rarely anyone asks a nurse how she/he is. Nurses work crazy long hours and they are often overwhelmed. They leave their kids for great stretches of time, they rarely get enough sleep. They deserve some attention and you can end up having a good conversation that can distract you from your own drama.

A good relationship with your nurse is your key to a bearable stay in the hospital. They are the ones who can get you a vase for the flowers or can get you a painkiller when something is throbbing and all the doctors have gone home. They can make concessions for you. I had a lovely nurse who switched all the generic pictures in my room with the ones in the hallway and other rooms, because I was desperate to look at seascapes for three days rather than close-ups of flowers.

If you have to go back and forth to the hospital, you will see the same nurses over and over again, so it's worth it to get to know them. The nurses are your friends.

Often, when you ask a nurse a question about your condition, she/he won't tell you the answer because only the doctor is really allowed to discuss your case, due to confidentiality or maybe insurance liability. But if you do get on well with your nurses, they will have lots of useful information for you, especially because they've dealt with lots of people who've had similar situations.

Smile and look every person who helps you in the eye. Everyone. From the guy emptying the rubbish bins to the cleaning crew to the doctors. They are human, too.

The one compliment I can give Memorial Sloan Kettering is that they had the best nurses ever. The hospital really is pleasant, clean, and extremely well-organized. One might not always agree with the treatment methods, but it is very well run and there is a nice view from the windows.

Your ROOMMATE

If you've really warmed up to a nurse, they might arrange it so you always have a private room. But sometimes it's just a very busy time and it's not possible.

If you have to share your room with another patient, be neighborly and considerate. Ask if it bothers them if you leave your toiletries on the bathroom counter. Introduce them to your visitors—or have your visitors be especially quiet if your roommate is trying to rest. I used to give my roommates a heads-up, i.e., "my daughters are coming at 2 pm, I hope they're not too noisy for you." If you can walk around, take those noisy guests out of your room. Unless of course, your roommate is enjoying their company, too!

Sometimes your roommate wants to talk, sometimes they just want to close their eyes and rest. If you have the energy, take a moment to be human and ask your roommate how she/he is feeling.

If you're more mobile than your roommate, ask if she/he needs help. Sometimes, it's just nice to have someone else there.

PART TWO:

It's still a hideous proposition if you must stay in hospital, but there are ways you can make it more bearable, maybe even pleasant. Sometimes it's as easy as a list of things that you might bring, or have friends or relatives bring, that makes it feel more homey.

Your DECOR

If you have to go to the hospital regularly, like for chemo once a week, try and always bring some fresh flowers with you when you check in. You can't always count on friends and visitors to bring you flowers and it's so nice to have a bit of nature in the room. Again, if your treatment makes you (or your roommate) feel queasy around certain scents, skip flowers that have a fragrance.

I always get flowers because it makes the smell of rubbing alcohol and chemicals less omnipresent. Unfortunately, even if you get lilies, peonies, or roses, they aren't that fragrant on the East coast of the U.S. because hot house flowers don't often have a strong scent. However, if you have a roommate, I'd skip paperwhites or narcissus or jasmine because they do get strong. But even unscented flowers or greens are better than nothing.

They say an experience of nature is calming and clears the head but you can't really bring a forest or a meadow in there. When things are tense, you can gaze at the life and light surging through those bright green leaves and petals and feel a little transported.

Be considerate of your roommate though. If he or she is feeling ill, you might have to move the flowers out of range or take them away all together.

I also brought a deep purple cashmere throw that my sister-in-law Soraya Sultan gave me. It covered the twin bed perfectly. It changed the color scheme from beige and white and those weird prints that are on hospital upholstery to something more cheerful. It was cozy. Sometimes those cotton blankets feel thin and ineffective. At other times, they get weird and tangled and sticky and you can't seem to get them in a comfortable place.

I once brought in a Diptyque scented candle. The nurse kindly let me light it for about a minute. I had to immediately blow it out because it could have exploded the oxygen tanks in the wall (who knew?) In any case, scented candles are out. If you don't have a sickly roommate, diptyque makes a scented hanging thing—figuer—which is something fresh and faint that almost everyone likes and it never smells artificial to me.

Your ENTERTAINMENT

You could bring in a CD player but if you had a roommate who hated Mozart, you would have to use headphones. I brought my laptop, headphones, and a lot of really silly comedy DVDs. Since chemo made me spacey and stupid, I watched ridiculous things with lots of slapstick and simple storylines (my mind wandered like crazy). Laughter is known to increase the strength of your immune system and they passed time.

I didn't bring books or even fashion magazines since it was difficult to read. The chemo also made me dizzy and I couldn't focus on the page, all the words turned into little rows of ants.

Your SNACKS

Bringing your own snacks is key. When I was having chemo, I was trying desperately to change my diet to lots of organic vegetables, phytonutrient live foods, and anti-oxidants. Also, let's face it, the food is horrendous in almost any hospital. I wanted something that had a taste and a texture, too.

I recommend eating organic even more emphatically while you're having chemo or radiation or surgery. Your body is already being bombarded by chemicals, toxins, and shock. It needs to be fed and nurtured gently.

Also, hospitals give you food at meal times and it takes forever from the time you've asked for it 'til it gets there. And once you're hooked up to the I.V., it's a drag to get around. If you're likely to be hungry before or after meals, it is wise to bring snacks.

Personally, I liked Brad's Raw Kale Chips, Nasty Hot. I buy them by the case since you save about $2.00 a box that way. I found chemo made me crave sharp, strong tastes. The sharp bite and crispy texture battled the nausea (which comes back just thinking about it). Also, bring some snacks that you can put in that big drawer beside the bed. That way you can get them yourself without having to ask anyone or having to unplug and push your stupid I.V. all the way down the wall as you try and find the kitchen. Tortilla chips. Raw almonds. Dried fruit.

What I did keep in the fridge were a box or two of fresh, organic blueberries, and some almond or coconut milk. I could add the fruit and nut milk to oatmeal in the morning for breakfast or put the milk in my tea. Any time anyone came over I'd ask them to bring me a fresh-pressed green vegetable juice from the local juice bar rather than chocolates.

I'd also ask for salads a lot, but later on in chemo, I found it hard to chew rough pieces of lettuce with all the sores in my mouth. If I was really nauseated, tiny bits of iceberg lettuce made me feel better. Ice water was good for that, too.

Last of all, it's nice to have something to offer your guests if people come and visit you. I'd bring some organic rice crackers and maybe even cookies or chips for my kids. Though, most people are so creeped out by being in the hospital setting that they decline any snacks at all.

Given the ubiquity of staph and other bacteria in hospital settings, it might be wiser not to let anyone else eat there.

Your NECESSITIES:

An EYEMASK is key. A nice silk one or an organic cotton one. They NEVER turn the lights out in the hospital. I found I needed one with an elastic band so it stayed on my head when I finally fell asleep and flipped over. If it's pretty, even better. Sometimes it feels good to have something really nice to look at. It makes you feel glamorous.

Last of all, sometimes chemo makes your eyes burn and it feels nice to have a cool eye mask against your skin.

A LONG SWEATER, dressing gown or sweatshirt with a zip or button front makes a huge difference because those stupid hospital gowns open in the back. I preferred a big cotton surfer's sweatshirt because the bright blue color cheered me up and the cotton was super soft and beat-up. It was the length of a coat so I could close it up and look less like an invalid (or so I thought) when I wandered the hallways. And since it was cotton, I could fall asleep with it on and not get uncomfortably hot in the night. What you have to remember is, whatever you're wearing on your top when you get the I.V. put in is what you'll be stuck in for the next two or three days until they take it out (because of the sleeves). So choose wisely. Dress for comfort as well as style.

Personally, I hated those blue-and-white printed hospital gowns that looked like they turned everyone into babies or sick people. I liked being able to cover mine up and be an individual. I somehow found it easier to muster up some dignity whilst speaking to the doctors on their rounds if I looked like a normal person. More on that later...

SLIPPERS. Basically, you have to go from your bed to the bathroom repeatedly and you don't want to do it in your socks and then put them back in your bed. Socks also feel really awful if you step in something slightly wet. I recommend hard-soled slippers, like the kind that you can walk your dog in or wear to go get the newspaper in the morning. In the winter, Uggs shearling scuffs are nice, though the pastel colors get dirty really fast. I was lucky enough to have a pair of very brightly colored Birkenstocks and I always got fresh pedicures before I came in because it cheered me up to look at my feet. They were the only part of body that stayed recognizable through everything.

WIPES. I liked some natural lavender wipes. They are good to wipe your hands before you eat or to wipe off your tray if you want to put your laptop on it. They leave a fresh scent behind. You can also touch them to your temples when the doctor has just left. When things feel dire, the smell of lavender clears your head.

All this stuff may seem absurdly expensive given your circumstances, but I suggest you invest in it anyway. It makes you feel chic and aristocratic and helps you continue to behave in a "noblesse oblige" fashion. In the end, the way you treat the people who help you will make all the difference.

This is one tip that won't practically affect the tone of your stay, but it will ease your mind and help you feel like you are part of the process.

PART THREE:

Make friends with the DOCTORS.

As my friend Sancha Mandy reminded me, they come in packs. The worst time (for me) was the morning rounds. Because they would be fresh and dressed and joking and chatting amongst themselves as they came in. Then you feel like a feeble, unwashed, beat-up vagrant who hasn't slept all night (because they wake you up every two or three hours to check your vitals) and—as I explained about the sleeves, if you have an I.V., you're either dressed like a baby in those unflattering blue-and-white flower printed gowns or you've been sleeping in your clothes for a couple of days. It doesn't help that the doctors all talk about you in the third-person.

Here's a strategy that worked for me. I woke up (like I was ever REALLY asleep) an hour or two before rounds.

I'd get the nurse to unhook my I.V. and I'd attempt a shower or sponge bath in the bathroom. I'd change to a freshly-laundered gown. Then I'd brush my hair and teeth, put on mascara and blush and attempt to look as civilized and lucid as possible. I put my hair (while I still had some) in a ponytail. When I got back to bed, I'd get out my laptop and run through all the questions I'd had.

The doctors would come in then. Usually it's the big honcho, the head of the department, surrounded by fawning student-interns and a couple of nurses. The main doctor prods and pokes you in embarrassing ways and then the young doctors-in-training all ask if they can, too, just to further humiliate you. In order to maintain a sense of dignity, I suggest you take the time to learn as many of their names as you can. Then have a bright conversation with them about your condition. Take back the situation. They become less invasive and treat you more as a person, albeit a bald, skinny one.

Remember, this is about you as a human being, not you as a science project. This is the key moment to ask your doctor every single question you have about your treatment. She/he will do their absolute best to answer you because they are also training all these young doctors and want to show good bedside manner to them. If there is something you don't like or that is not working, this is the time to ask.

Make sure to do your research first and keep your questions on point so the doctors have to answer specifically rather than in vague generalizations. If you start to learn some medical jargon, i.e. "I feel pressure in the lower left quadrant of my abdomen," so much the better. They treat you even more respectfully.

If you find something that makes you question a specific part of your treatment, print it out (but not massive texts with pages and pages) and give it to your doctor. Most doctors work hard and lead somewhat harried lives. They can't always keep up with the latest information.

I've spoken to doctors who say the internet has done a disservice to patients because "they all think they are experts." I suppose you could diagnose yourself with all kinds of diseases and freak yourself out no end if you are that kind of worried, hypochondriac-type person.

When I was in high school, one of my best friends (who used to keep a personal stash of antibiotics in his cupboard) had a father who was a doctor. He used to joke, "The first thing a doctor always says? Never self-medicate."

There is certainly a truth in that one shouldn't be taking antibiotics and OTC crap wildly.

However, what doctors sometimes forget is that you ARE an expert in one thing: your own body—and the body of your young child. You are the only one who knows how you feel. Your intuition—if you take the time to listen to it—will probably tell you what's really wrong.

Whatever happens in the hospital, remember that this particular movie is all about you. Be kind to others but don't forget one thing: Treat yourself like the hero that you are.

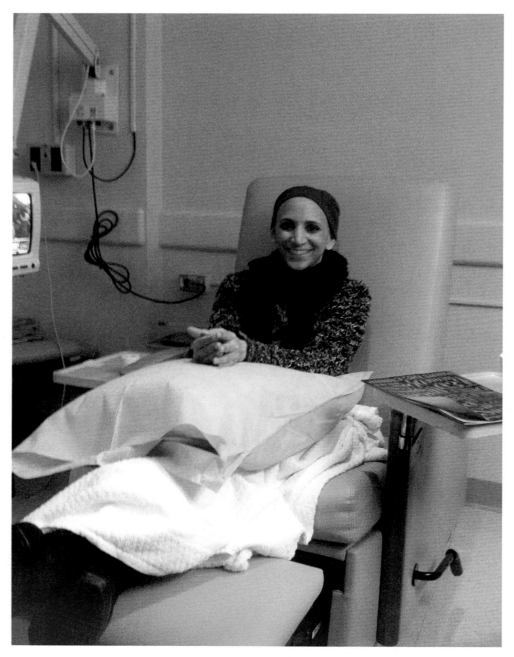

Getting chemotherapy and planning my skincare.

Beauty and Cancer

Skin products
that don't irritate supersensitive cheeks.
Super gentle prettiness for hairless people.

CHAPTER FIVE: The Beauty of Cancer

This may sound all superficial when you are in what feels like a life or death situation, but beauty products are actually crucial. Scientific studies show that when you are happier, you heal faster. But also, when you look better, people treat you differently. We are only human.

I felt hideous when everything started falling apart, not least because people would stare (just for a minute and then look away). I looked like a scrawny, hairless alien. I don't know if they thought I had cancer or something else, but people tended to give me a wide berth, as though my disease just might be catching. My daughters gave me a gift certificate to a place called Spa Castle—a gigantic Korean spa with all kinds of relaxing treatments— and I didn't go because I thought everyone would REALLY stare at me in a bathing suit. It didn't help that most massage therapists, nail salons, aestheticians, even dentists would refuse me treatment because they were scared of what the cancer might do—or my compromised immune system.

Friends would say, "You look great!" in a loudish, fakely cheerful voice. Or they'd tell me about someone else who had chemo and looked much worse. I ran errands, worked, and was happy that I could, but I felt embarrassed about my looks. I went to see one of my daughters in her school play and, between scenes, I came out into the lobby and sat on the floor and cried because I felt like a leper.

I was in a meeting at an ad agency pitching, of all things, a hair care line, and feeling totally awkward. I mentioned to the table that I didn't need shampoo. My boss laughed, "No, you need Miracle-Gro!" Well, that broke the tension.

So.

How you look matters.

If you are reading this for a friend or family member who is sick, keep that in mind.

To start out, let's forget serious beauty treatments and think about discomfort. Your skin feels rough, hot, dry and itchy—or some combination of the three—during chemo and/or radiation. Unfortunately, almost any commercial product you apply will irritate the skin even further. Your eyes are often red, dry and swollen.

First things first, I didn't use any cleansers at all. My skin was just too dry. I rinsed it with water. If I attempted to use anything even slightly exfoliating, it made my cheeks sting. I only wore natural make-up products so I didn't need to remove them. If I really felt I needed a cleanse, I actually splashed unsweetened kombucha tea on my face!

For moisturizer, some people suggest you splash water on your face and then apply a thin layer of sweet almond oil. This is the most basic level of care but it is best for babies with eczema because their skin is naturally plump, hydrated and soft. Oil helps seal the moisture into your skin, but it doesn't give your skin the cooling, soothing, quenching it craves.

During my 25+ years in the beauty industry, I used to joke that all the expensive skin creams worked about as well as Crisco with fragrance and a nice jar. This is not fair and not totally true.

Even post-chemo, what your skin needs is a three-part solution:

1. An emollient
2. A humectant
3. An occlusive

Many skin products incorporate the three, but it can be better to do each one well.

The emollient is a moisturizer. It hydrates, softens, and plumps up the fine lines. It feels good on the skin. The reason you can't rely on it alone is that it evaporates very quickly. Thus it can leave the skin feeling even dryer than it did to begin with.

Next, you need a humectant. Humectants draw the moisture from the air into your skin. Glycerin, coconut oil, and hyaluronic acid (sounds scary but it's actually something your body creates to lubricate itself) are humectants. If you use too much of a humectant, your skin looks dewy, but can feel sticky to the touch, especially as the product dries - because it does dry - into a thick gel.

Thus top it all off, you need an occlusive. An occlusive seals in the moisture and protects and fortifies your skin's moisture barrier. The moisture on your skin not only makes the skin softer and more resilient, it creates a barrier to bacteria, environmental irritants and pollutants. That's why dry skin is actually more prone to infection.

For me, the best moisturizer during chemo was a simple Calendula cream. Look for organic, natural brands like Weleda or California Baby. Make sure it is unscented. Calendula cooled the skin and soothed the itchy red rash. I still travel with a tube of this as my face is very sensitive to stress and different kinds of water. (Personally, after cleansing, I start with a vitamin C product to help re-build the collagen, reduce the dark spots and splotches you get from chemotherapy, and brighten the skin. Be careful with this though, as the wrong product can irritate the skin and cause MORE redness (and that's hardly what you need). Liquid Gold is the only brand I recommend for people with cancer, since it's natural and designed for sensitive skin.)

Then I used a humectant. My friend Ruba Abu Nimah was working for Estee Lauder at the time. She sent me the Creme De La Mer serum, a rich gel fortified with seaweed or algae—that, unlike most commercially-prepared products, didn't have a heavy scent or color. Today, I use a pure hyaluronic acid and natural plant stem cell combination and a natural rosewater and glycerin mist. My favorite is Liquid Gold cell quench which is made of hyaluronic acid and plant stem cells. I spray on some rosewater and glycerin and then roll on a little cell quench and spread it around with my finger tips.

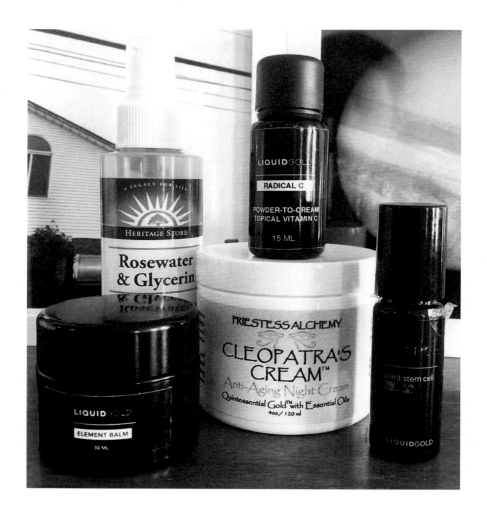

My fave beauty products for people in treatment—and my routine today.

For my occlusive, I then used a heavy moisturizer with a sweet almond oil base called Cleopatra's cream. It's made by a friend of natural, non-GMO ingredients—including antibacterial coconut oil and homeopathic suspensions of minerals and seems to be the ONLY thing that really hydrates my post-chemo dryness. It still smells lovely but not fake in anyway.

Last, I topped it with a balm or oil at night. I've seen herbal shops selling calendula balms made of herbal extracts and essential oils. As long as it is not too scented, you could use that instead. I would test it on your arm and see how it feels. I use Weleda's Skin Food or The Liquid Gold's balm with vitamin E that is great for sealing in the moisture and healing. When you wake up in the morning, your skin is baby-soft.

Finally, remember that the moisture comes from the inside, too. While you are having chemo, drink water like crazy and make sure you are getting your good fats—avocados, coconut oil, nuts, rice bran oil. I took four capsules a day of rice bran oil, two capsule of rosemary oil, and four capsules a day of seabuckthorn oil.

Everything you apply to your skin gets absorbed into your blood stream, so if you wouldn't eat it, you probably shouldn't rub it into your face, especially when you are weak and your immune system is compromised. Do your research and buy products that are organic, natural and free of endocrine-interrupting chemicals – including their containers!

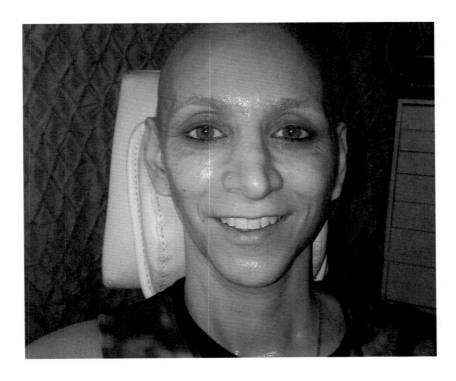

One month after I stopped chemotherapy.

My face well moisturized—just eyeliner but nothing else!

When you are all greased-up, let it soak in for a little while so that you don't look too slippery. Then it's time for make-up! There is a little-known brand called Illuminare which was actually designed to be super gentle for a breast cancer patient and is made out of natural minerals. It's a make-up artist's secret, as it blends really well, a teensy bit goes a long way, and it is non-irritating, even if you fall asleep with it on. Since it has a high mineral content, it works as a sunscreen as well—very useful since the skin becomes very photosensitive during chemotherapy and radiation—and it actually helps your skin heal.

Illuminare makes eye products that do not irritate the eyes (but irritatingly, require separate brushes—though that forces you to clean them often which is good) and nontoxic lip colors that last all day. One finds that one's lips not only get dry and cracked, they become pale.

I still wore my kajal every single day, unless my eyes got too prickly. Kajal is a South Asian eyeliner made of charcoal and healing oils. I use a brand called Hashmi Kajal. It's supposedly made out of Ayurvedic ingredients and protects your eyesight. It didn't bother my eyes, it's cheap and the only bad thing about it is that the plastic cap is really cheap and can break off in your bag and smear the waterproof stuff everywhere so keep it in a ziplock bag. I rinsed it in cold water between uses.

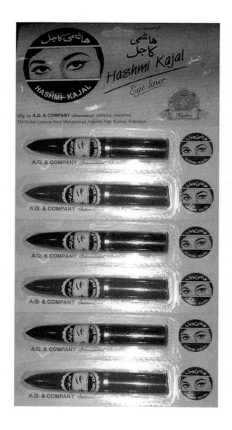 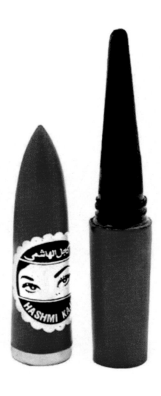

Apart from kajal, I am sucky at applying make-up myself but there are a million great tutorials on youtube. Watch them but, be supercareful with the products you choose. It is not worth the discomfort of skin and eyes that are even more irritated than before. I tried my daughters' make-up and came home and cried again because of how much they made my eyes sting and my face hurt.

My friend Mary Schook showed me how to safely apply false lashes if I needed to go out. And these days, there are no shortage of brow products (it's amazing how weird people look with no eyebrows).

Brush color on your brows—or where they were—slightly lighter than you think because it can very quickly make you look mad. When you first start, ask someone else to make sure you haven't turned yourself into Salvador Dali or Lucille Ball in the early 60s.

Most people undergoing cancer treatments become very slim. If you were never slim before, here is your chance to try layering! I'd recommend choosing fabrics that are very smooth and soft so as not to irritate your skin further. I used to start with a very thin, soft cotton t-shirt underneath everything. I also found that a thin pair of cotton leggings under a loose shirt or dress were useful, because there were so many instances during treatment where one had to undress one part of the body or another. With layers like that, you could reveal an arm, a hand, a foot, or a leg without leaving the rest of yourself exposed. That way, you feel like you maintain a level of dignity.

Since I live in New York City AND I didn't want to have to buy an entirely new wardrobe before, during and after treatment, I chose most stuff in neutral colors - black, white and gray - with accents in red, blue or neon orange. I added a bright pop of color near the face, a scarf or hat, to cheer myself up.

When it comes to your treatment, ask your oncologist if you can avoid the prednisone or steroids. They give the steroids along with the cancer treatment for a few different reasons, one is to reduce swelling—especially if you have a brain tumor or a tumor that is blocking your basic life functions, i.e., digestion or absorption or elimination of nutrients. If you have a cancer in your breast, uterus, or another area, you might find that the reason they are giving you steroids is to reduce the nausea or give you energy when the chemo drugs weaken you. The side effect of prednisone for many people is puffiness and weight gain and in the long run, thinning of skin and bones. I decided not to take any.

The chemo nurse said that, as a small person, if I was concerned about osteoporosis in the long term, then avoiding the steroids might be a good idea—"If you can manage the nausea."

What I did instead of the steroids was take massive amounts of ginger. I took three to four ginger capsules—the Gaia ones—just before I was plugged into my chemo. I took a couple more any time I felt nauseated. I added fresh ginger root to my green juice and I added dried ginger and turmeric to anything I cooked. I still had a lot of nausea but never unmanageably so. I never vomited though I often didn't feel like eating.

Interestingly, new studies show that fasting during chemotherapy can actually make it more effective, so perhaps not eating and not feeling hungry is not a bad thing.

Fasting strengthens the immune system and helps the chemo (and body) differentiate between cancer cells and normal cells and it also makes radiation more effective.

Without the steroids, I felt exhausted after chemo. I needed to go home and sleep for several hours, which was probably very healing. Whereas my friends who did have the steroids found themselves up at night vacuuming the living room and scrubbing the bathtubs.

In other words, the short term effects of steroids—puffiness, weight gain, bloating—and the long term effects—thinning of the skin and weakening of the bones—might make you consider removing them from your regimen. Do your own research. Then ask your oncologist or chemo or radiation nurse if it is possible—and how one might mitigate the side effects of your treatment without them.

I recommend checking on the long term side effects of each of the drugs in your regimen and protocol and see what you might do to reduce them, for instance, how to protect your heart and your liver and kidneys.

In terms of fragrance, when you really look odd, it's nice to smell sweet. A lot of people find that chemotherapy and/or radiation makes them nauseated and sensitive to smells, especially artificial ones. I found that, at my most nauseated, the scent of natural grapefruit oil was fresh and clean smelling. Lavender and rosemary—but the natural oils, not the fake stuff—have a green, camphorousness that can cut through the nausea. They are both also calming and antibacterial. Personally, I also found natural rose and jasmine oils very soothing as well as sexy (and not much made me feel sexy at that time).

My suggestion is to go to health food store or natural aromatherapy place and test out some of the oils, or ask people to bring you a few. Try a tiny bit on your wrist and leave it on for a while. Or put it on a sweater or sweatshirt. See if it smells nice or it makes you feel sick as the day goes on. If you can't handle any scented products at all, don't worry about it. But given the hormonal and other nasty effects of synthetic fragrance, I'd recommend you avoid them all together.

Also, look at the products in your bathroom. Shampoos, conditioners, body wash, soaps, and lotions can all irritate the skin and eyes—and they also penetrate the skin and enter the bloodstream. I would go as natural as you can manage. I used Dr. Bronner's Lavender soap (I didn't need shampoo), a natural toothpaste with no fluoride (another possible carcinogen), and food grade sweet almond oil or coconut oil on my body after bathing. Then I rubbed on a little natural flower oil. I used Weleda's Rose deodorant and it seemed to work well.

If you are getting radiation, I recommend a 20-30 minute soak in one cup of epsom salt, one cup of baking soda, and one cup of natural sea salt after treatment. It both calms and remineralizes your body while it helps you release the radiation. Take a shower afterwards.

I made a big effort to reduce my use of plastic bottles and artificial cleaning products. All my years of swimming laps made me adore the chlorine smell of Clorox Clean-Up and bleach. But you can get much less toxic cleaners made of hydrogen peroxide and they are just as effective at killing germs.

I did not wear a wig because I found them itchy, expensive, and ugly. (Plus, I have fond memories of Sinead O'Connor and the model Eve as bad ass b@#ches.) Since I underwent chemotherapy from October 'til February, I was partial to some extremely soft cashmere beanies made by Meg Cohen. These are the nicest, thickest cashmere I have ever felt and they are locally-made by the nicest person. It's a tiny business that behaves with the best ethics.

Think about it this way, if you are going to have something close to your skin (and your crown chakra), make sure it has good energy!

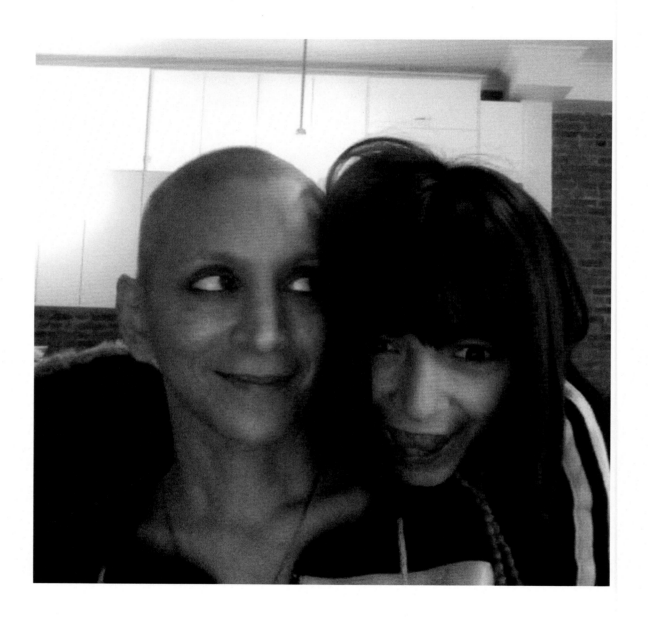

Trust and Medicine

How faith in your cure
and yourself helps.

CHAPTER SIX: Trust and Healing

The biggest problem right now in the medical industry and the healing community is trust. It's also keeping us from getting well. You can't focus on getting healthy if you don't have faith in the cure or your own ability to recover or you don't believe your practitioner. As any hypnotist or meditation teacher will tell you, the best way to change your world is to change how you feel about it.

People don't trust doctors, what with all the news about kickbacks from pharmaceutical companies (check out the dollars for docs site to see if yours has), doctors working 24 hours a day because insurance companies squeeze their time (thus sometimes they make mistakes), more doctors and nurses handing off patients in shorter shifts and the horrible instances where the process goes wrong and a person gets hurt.

Every day, I seem to get another piece of direct mail/email with a headline like

"WHAT DOCTORS AREN'T TELLING YOU" or

" WHAT THE MEDICAL INDUSTRY DOESN'T WANT YOU TO KNOW..."

Doctors don't trust patients, because medicine is imperfect. Doctors are humans and doing the best they can, and patients are likely to sue them if the insurance companies don't do it first. Mainstream doctors don't trust alternative health practitioners because they've never learned what they do.

In the complementary medicine community, many energy healers, acupuncturists, homeopaths, naturopaths, and massage therapists don't trust each other's work and they really don't trust the allopathic doctors.

And average people don't know if they can trust the alternative medical practitioners because the government has cracked down so hard on them, they can barely hang a shingle, let alone help anyone in any way. I was talking to Tracy Beers who is a very successful hypnotist, especially working with cancer patients. She survived cancer herself so she knows the drill. I asked her what she says when people ask for a guarantee—like what if the treatment doesn't get them to quit smoking (or lose weight or whatever it is)?

She said, "Does your doctor give you a guarantee? Does he guarantee the penicillin will work?"

And I thought about it and mumbled something about test results, but of course, we all know that about scientists falsifying research.

Not only does my doctor NOT guarantee results, if something doesn't work or has horrid side-effects, I have to contact her and pay for all the different tests and other prescriptions that she guinea-pigs me on, along with all the subsequent appointments.

One thing I have discovered in being ill is that one needs an arsenal of healers. We need allopathic, regular doctors, and internists and surgeons who can set a broken bone or stitch one's face back together after a taxi accident (like mine back in 2011).

We need energy healers who can help our body's own healing system work better and help us re-gain our spirit. Acupuncturists who can make sure the systems are running properly. Nutritionists and naturopaths who can help us eat well enough that our wounds disappear. Homeopaths who can help with the swelling and speed the recovery. Some good friends who can help us do some research and find a lawyer and make sure we don't miss the deadline to sue the taxi company, (I did, you only have 30 days, but I questioned the litigious society we've created and the poor taxi driver looked terrified and sorrowful.)

Personally, I don't trust *anyone* to do it alone. (Except myself and Universal Intelligence or God—and even that's a team.)

As humans, we need to stop expecting easy answers. There is no single way to address any challenge. And no one should expect perfect solutions from any one practitioner. We need a team, we need ourselves (because NOTHING will work unless you want it and believe it and are willing to put your own work in too).

And if our practitioners don't feel safe with us—trust me, they are terrified—they can't really help us.

So drink your green juice and a lot more water. Stop the junk food. When you are trying to heal a systemic illness, step away from the lawyers and spend more time opening up to your healers—on all sides of the spectrum. Cut them some slack. Take some responsibility for yourself.

You will feel better.

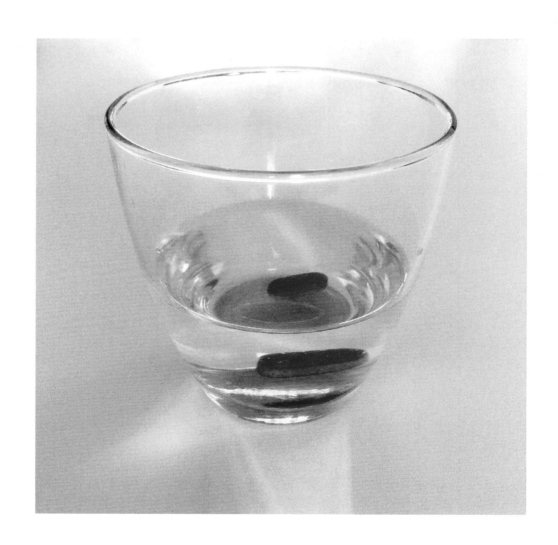

All Those Pills!

The Supplements I took – during,
after and in lieu of traditional treatment.

CHAPTER SEVEN: All Those PILLS! Supplements I Took and What Might Work for You.

I was watching *Family Guy* (the Amazons were watching, actually) and Brian (the dog) had fallen in love with an older woman. Stewie is the brilliant baby.

The dialogue went like this:

Stewie Griffin: Hey its 4:30. Isn't there an early bird special you should be running off to?

Brian Griffin: She's 50, Stewie she's not an old woman [*His phone rings and he takes it out and answers it*] Hello?... Hey Rita... [*His smile turns to a frown and he talks with a hushed voice*]... uh, no I'm not hungry yet... well, if we get there by 5:30 I'm sure they'll honor it...

Stewie Griffin: Brian, is she calling dinner "supper?"

Brian Griffin: [*Still on the phone*] So, uh—what're ya doing this afternoon?

Stewie Griffin: [*Imitating an elderly woman's voice*] Oh I'm just sorting out my pills for the week, sweetie.

Brian Griffin: [*Still on the phone*] Well, you do that, and I'll be over a little later. [He hangs up the phone]

Stewie Griffin: [*Condescending noise*] Did I get it? Was she sorting out her pills for the week? That little plastic thing with the seven boxes? [*Excited noise*]

Brian Griffin: Actually, she just got back from the gym and she's jumping in the shower.

Stewie Griffin: ... she got a chair in that shower?

Brian Griffin: Shut up! [*He leaves*]

I am officially an old woman. Since my first appointment with Integrative Oncologist Mitchell Gaynor, I got one of those plastic pill boxes, along with an entire tray full of bottles of supplements. The supplements were put together by him and a genius pharmacist called David Restrepo and a very good Drugless Practitioner/Acupuncturist called Galina Semyonova. If you have any health issues at all, I suggest talking to someone who knows supplements as there is a lot one can rebalance with vitamins, minerals, oils, herbs, and enzymes.

After three years of studying Chinese medicine, Holistic Nutrition, and North American Herbology, everyone asks me about supplements—but they rarely take them. Or they buy a few from the drugstore and then forget to take them.

The main obstacles to successful supplementation are as follows:

1. Knowing which brands provide the most bio-available (usable for your body) sources and forms

2. How much to take and when to take them, for your own body.

3. Whether you take them with or without food and what time of day.

4. Which supplements work better in tandem and which you should never have together. and

5. Waiting to feel the effects. Patience! Herbs, homeopathic medicines, and vitamins work gently—it can take up to 6 weeks to feel the results ¬– which is the goal.

Natural medicines are meant to work in tandem with your body to address the underlying causes of your issues. In the beginning, they might give you an upset stomach or a headache, so you should have your practitioner's number on hand in case you need to have the dose adjusted for you. Generally, you should wait at least two weeks before you take a bigger dose and six weeks before you decide they are not working.

It's like exercise. The first day you go for a run, you will not drop an inch from your waist. Maybe even if you run every day for a week, you might feel more energized, but you still won't be much skinnier. Real change takes time. Rushing it can make you sick. Imagine if you immediately started running five miles a day after not doing any exercise for years, you'd probably feel pretty bad and more than likely you would injure yourself.

Here's the other argument I hear against supplementation:

> "I get all the vitamins and minerals I need from my food and most doctors say that's enough."

There are several reasons why relying solely on food doesn't work for most people—but especially not people with cancer. The food we eat is of varying quality, depending on how and where it was grown, how it was transported, how long it hung out in the shop and then your fridge, and how you cooked it. Basically, the vitamin and mineral content is dropping since it gets pulled off the stalk. And we're not even talking about how much less nutritious conventionally grown food is than organic. Then, depending on what's going on with your body, you can't always ingest all the nutrients in your food. Especially, as you get older, and your body produces fewer enzymes and acids to break the food down, you don't get the same value.

Last, if you have cancer or another disease, you know it is systemic. Cancer makes your body weak and it also can take away your appetite and limit your ability to absorb the nutrition from your food, so you need more vitamins and minerals than you can possibly get from eating. If you are getting chemo or radiation, even more reason to supplement to help your good cells stay strong during the onslaught.

Obstacle five is the reason I never take multivitamins. First, because the various vitamins might cancel each other out, next because there might be things in the combination that my body doesn't need. Also, some substances are best absorbed by your body at night and others in the morning. It's like the shampoo-conditioner-in-one, they never seem to do especially well at either job. Admittedly, a multi is better than nothing. So, if that's your starting point:

Chop Your Multivitamin in Half!

If you do take a multivitamin, some advice. Choose one that comes in smaller capsules so that you can divide the dose, take half of the dose—or chop the pill in half and take half—in the morning, with/after breakfast and half mid-afternoon or after lunch. The reason is that your body can use the vitamins most effectively with food—your stomach secretes hydrochloric acid to digest food which breaks down the supplement and allows absorption (otherwise, the supplement can go straight out to your vitamin-enriched urine) and it can spread out the effects throughout the day.

Drop a Test Pill in a Glass of Water

Also, with any supplement you buy, try to choose capsules or liquid forms rather than pills. This is because the glue they use to bind pills is often so strong, even your stomach acids can't break it apart. To test if the pill will break down once you swallow it, drop one in a glass of water and see how long it takes to disintegrate. If it takes more than an hour, the pill is probably going straight through your body undigested.

If you only take a few supplements, Dr. Oz recommends these five supplements: a multivitamin, calcium and magnesium combination, vitamin D3, omega-3 (or fish oil) and folic acid. A multi is better than taking no supplements at all. But I disagree with the folate, unless you are likely to become pregnant. I would take a B-vitamin combination that I mention later in the chapter.

The amount you need of vitamins and minerals depends on your body. Sometimes you will need less, sometimes in larger amounts, sometimes not at all. Personally, I didn't take vitamin A or B, because my body didn't need it—though now I do—perhaps I was getting enough from dietary sources. I take more D3 in the winter when I am not exposed to enough sunlight and less in the summer when I am outside a lot.

If you have cancer, there was an oncologist called Nicholas Gonzalez who used pancreatic enzymes to fight the growth. This therapy is based on the assumption that cancer cells have a thick coating that makes them invisible to your immune system. That keeps your body from attacking them. Otherwise strong immune-boosting supplements, like turmeric and quercetin, can't get through. The pancreatic enzymes digest/melt away the coating on the cancer cells, allowing your body to then destroy them naturally. While most young people produce pancreatic enzymes sufficiently, when you have cancer, you REALLY need them, thus supplementation can be key. I did not see Dr. Gonzalez, but I did take 15 capsules of pancreatic enzymes, three or four times daily.

Check Where the Vitamin/Mineral/Herb Comes From

With calcium supplements, one has to be careful about the source of the calcium. Many inexpensive supplements are made from ground up seashells or limestone. These substances are full of calcium but they are not always "bio-available," meaning, your body can't use them properly. Again, off to the kidneys, where they might cause stones. Also, without sufficient amounts of magnesium, vitamin D3, and vitamin K, too much calcium can cause an imbalance in your body, effectively draining calcium from your bones into your blood stream and soft tissues where, again, they can block arteries and cause trouble.

The best way to get calcium that is both soluble (dissolves in stomach acids) and is used by your body (bioavailable) is through plants and sea vegetables and algae. I suggest you look for a supplement that includes magnesium, vitamin K, D3, and strontium. Personally, when I do take calcium, I take New Chapter Bone Health and I break up the dose (six small pills) throughout the day. I take the majority of the pills at bedtime because it makes me calmer and helps me sleep better.

Similarly, many vitamin E and D3 supplements are made of soybean oil. Soybean oil goes rancid very quickly, which makes it toxic. While soy is a phytoestrogen and has become controversial as a food source, the main reason I don't eat it is that 98% of the soy produced in this country is GMO. I believe anyone who has had cancer should avoid GMOs.

Current recommendations for EVERYONE who is worried about getting cancer or bone loss supplement is at least 5,000 to 8,000 iu everyday. To figure out what that means, 15 to 20 minutes out in the sun in Cape Cod gives you about 25,000 iu. Xymogen makes a good one that includes K2, which has the added advantage of being good for your teeth. Personally, I take four to six drops every day of Micellized Vitamin D3. Along with large doses of vitamin C, it has also been shown to reduce asthma attacks in children. And taking regular supplements of D3 can reduce your chance of cancer by 70%!

Ameena's Anti-Cancer Supplements Protocol:

[A disclaimer: I am NOT a doctor. I am telling you my own experience. Everything I list here, I tested on my body while still under the care of an oncologist at Memorial Sloan Kettering. My liver, kidneys, blood pressure, eyes, and skin texture all improved greatly while taking them during chemotherapy and afterwards.]

I TOOK THIS:

Turmeric, 300 mg, twice or three times daily. Curcumin is the active ingredient in Turmeric, so the one you take should have a high active curcumin value—read the label.

I took Meriva-SR by Thorne Encapsulations. I've recently learned that activating the cancer and inflammation-fighting effects of turmeric requires a fat or oil and black pepper. I have a friend I worked with who found that the most effective way to take turmeric was to put a heaping teaspoon of turmeric powder in a cup, mix in a tablespoon of coconut oil and a 1/4 teaspoon of black pepper and then gulp it down. She says it tastes nasty, but that's what is. Often when one isolates the active ingredient in a plant or a herb, it doesn't work as well. Most natural ingredients work better in their natural form.

Turmeric is good for inflammation of any sort so activated like that, it is also recommended for arthritis and I give it to my kids for headaches and cramps.

Alpha Lipoic Acid Sustain, 300 mg, once daily. I took Jarrow Brand. This helps reduce the irritation in your stomach. But the PolyMVA is a more bio-available form of this.

NAC, 600 mg, once daily. I took Pure Encapsulations. This increases your body's production of glutathione, which strengthen your nervous system and helps your body absorb other nutrients.

Rosemaria (rosemary oil) and Calendula, one capsules each, twice daily. I took Completely Green, but it was quite expensive so I switched to New Chapter's Omega 7, which has a combination of Rosemary and Calendula as well as Seabuckthorn. I currently take four capsules a day of New Chapter's Omega 7 which seems to hydrate my skin as well as help with my memory. From a herbalist P.O.V., rosemary is antibacterial but also a nerveine, it helps calm the spirit and reduce headaches.

Rice Bran Oil Tocotrienols, one capsule, twice daily. I took Pure Encapsulations. This is a non-soy vitamin E that hydrates the skin and organs but also fights free radicals, especially in breast cells.

Wheat Embryo, one capsules, twice daily. I took Completely Green, but there are others available. This is a rich oil that hydrates your skin beautifully, especially after chemo has ravaged it.

Plant-derived Calcium. I took Coxamin, one capsule, twice daily. Now I take the previously mentioned New Chapter Bone Health.

Vitamin D3, 8,000 iu. I took Micellized Vitamin D3, 1000 iu, eight drops daily in my green juice every morning.

Vitamin C, 1000 mg, three to four times daily. I used Lypospheric Vitamin C, I squeezed two envelopes in my green juice in the morning and one in the afternoon. I chose this brand because I noticed an immediate bounce in my energy levels after taking it. It's also recommended by the http://www.cancertutor.com/ website which is a not-for-profit resource for alternative/complementary cancer therapies. Whether or not you agree with Linus Pauling, vitamin C does seem to make you feel better—and if you take good quality l-ascorbic acid, you do not get an upset stomach or diarrhea when you take large quantities.

Shitake, one capsule, twice daily. I used Completely Green brand again. This was the brand recommended by Mitchell Gaynor. These days, I tend to take a multi-mushroom complex. I do, however, eat LOTS of mushrooms—Shitake, Maitaki, Reishi, Chanterelle. I was told no button, Portobello, or cremini mushrooms (which are all basically one kind of mushroom) because they are so watered-down that they have little to no nutritional value (the nutritionist I went to see, Joel Fuhrman, suggested they have negative value), however, it now seems that they are mildly beneficial anyway.

Pro-Omega, 1280 mg, one capsule, daily. This is one capsule of concentrated fish oil, manufactured by Nordic Naturals.

Peak Immune, 250 mg, two capsules, twice daily. This is a combination of rice bran and shitake polysaccharides (I think) and is designed for people with compromised immune systems. I did not take it again after the first four months after stopping chemotherapy.

Krill Oil, 500 mg, one capsule, twice daily. I don't know if it's redundant to take krill oil and fish oil but soon I didn't feel like I needed them both. I took the Mercola brand as I tend to find them trustworthy and conscious about their ingredients.

Immunotix 3-6, once daily. This is a beta-glucan which is especially useful for people who need more white blood cells and want to strengthen their bone marrow post-chemo. It is expensive and I only took it for three months.

Since I had neuropathy and balance and memory issues from the chemotherapy, I took several nerve formulas.

Alpha GPC, 300 mg, one capsule, twice daily. I took Jarrow brand. This is a phospholipid that crosses the brain barrier and helps learning and memory. My short-term still has some holes.

Co-Q 10, 200 mg, once daily. I buy my Co-q 10 in q-gel form from a company called epic4health. I have a friend whose father used to sell supplements and he recommended them as the best supplier of co-Q 10 and fish oil.

Enada, 5 mg, one capsule, twice daily. This is meant to improve mental clarity and energy. I took this for three months and then stopped as I wasn't sure what effect it had. Post-chemo, I had trouble with word retrieval, reading comprehension (big handicap for a copywriter), and short-term memory, which gave me terrible anxiety.

Rhodiola 60, one capsule, daily. I took Thorne Encapsulations brand. Rhodiola is an excellent anti-stress herb. I'd recommend it any time one is feeling overwhelmed or anxious and not getting enough rest. It helped a lot with the post-chemo hot flashes which were brought on by anxiety—and my constant confusion and memory issues. I found it very hard to understand the meaning of street signs or notices.

Triple-Bee Complex, one capsule, twice daily. This is a combination of bee pollen, royal jelly and propolis which are said to nourish the body and brain and activate killer cells. According to Mitchell Gaynor's *Cancer Prevention Program* book, out of print now, but a brilliant and useful text, bee pollen may delay or avert breast cancer. It's also great for seasonal allergies. The only place I disagree is his thoughts on soy.

Bacopa, one capsule, three times daily. This is an ayurvedic brain herb. Apparently, it is very useful to take for people who have Alzheimer's and/or Parkinson's. I did take it for some time but stopped as it no longer seemed useful. It is an adaptogen, meaning it will naturally adapt itself to your needs so one could take it in the long term.

Pancreatic Enzymes, 15 capsules, three times a day. I took the Allergy Research brand because they manufacture the capsules for Gonzalez.

Probiotics, three times daily. At first, I took 1/3 of a sachet of VSL3, the idea was to restore my digestive tract post-chemotherapy. Later, I wanted a larger selection of bacteria (for immune issues), so I started taking Mercola's Probiotic, which does not need to be refrigerated and is enteric-coated so it survives the trip through your intestines to your stomach.

PolyMVA, 2 tbsp, four times a day. This incredibly healing supplement is one the best cancer-killing products anywhere. They have thousands of testimonials on their site, and this supplement is especially good for the immune system, leukemia, and pancreatic cancer, as well as reducing the incidence of bone metastasis post-chemotherapy. Leukemia was the main side-effect of my chemo-drugs so I thought it wise. I have only caught one cold or flu in the past six years, even during the worst of my immune system damage post-chemotherapy. I am around lots of schoolchildren who cough, sneeze, share my food and drinks and wipe their noses on my towels. It's expensive but I recommend it to everyone who has cancer or even bad respiratory infections (at smaller doses).

Exhilarin, one pill, twice daily. This is an ayurvedic combination of herbs, including ashwaganda, holy basil, amla, and bacopa, which is very good for calm and focus, especially during menopause.

Resveratrol, 200 mg, once daily. I actually took Shaklee's Vivix which seemed to make an amazing difference in my skin quality, too. Sometimes, I switch it out with two capsules a day of Revgenetics Nitro 250.

Melatonin, 5 mg, two at bedtime daily. Personally, I found I built up too much of a tolerance to melatonin. I started needing 20 to 25 mg to fall asleep so I stopped and switched to a tea of chamomile, passionflower, valerian, skullcap, and hops.

Every afternoon, I drank one smoothie.
Here's the recipe:

- Delgado Protocol Stem Cell Strong, one scoop.
  This is a combination of mushrooms and fruits.
- 1/2 of an avocado
- 1 or 2 stalks of kale, deveined
- 1/2 cup of vanilla hemp milk
- A handful of fresh or frozen berries
- 1/2 cup of frozen acai
- Coconut water to make it more liquidy

Every morning, I drank a cup of hot water and lemon and then 16-24 oz of "green juice."
Here's my green juice recipe:

- 4 stalks of kale (deveined)
- 4 big leaves of romaine, swiss chard
  (or mustard greens – you might start to like the bitterness)
- 1/4 to 1/2 green apple
- 1/2 of a cucumber
- 3 to 4 stalks of celery
- 1 lemon
- 1 small bunch of parsley and/or coriander
- 1/4 to 1/2 inch of ginger root

Sometimes, I replaced the apple with carrot or radish, but carrots make the juice browner and radishes give it a bite – see what suits you.

Juicing is crucial when you have cancer because it floods your body with vitamins, minerals, and enzymes that are immediately available to your body. The proponents of juicing include Norman Walker, Max Gerson, Fred Bisci, Alex Junger, David Wolfe and a whole series of raw juice and food purveyors. There are a lot of juice recipes on their sites.

The best method for juicing is using a cold-press—at home, one can buy a Norwalk Juicer if one has a big kitchen—because it extracts the most nutrients with the least damage to the enzymes. Personally, I use the Omega VRT 350 slow juicer. If I don't have time, I buy my juice, but I make sure it is fresh, not hpp-processed and bottled for a month as that kills a lot of enzymes.

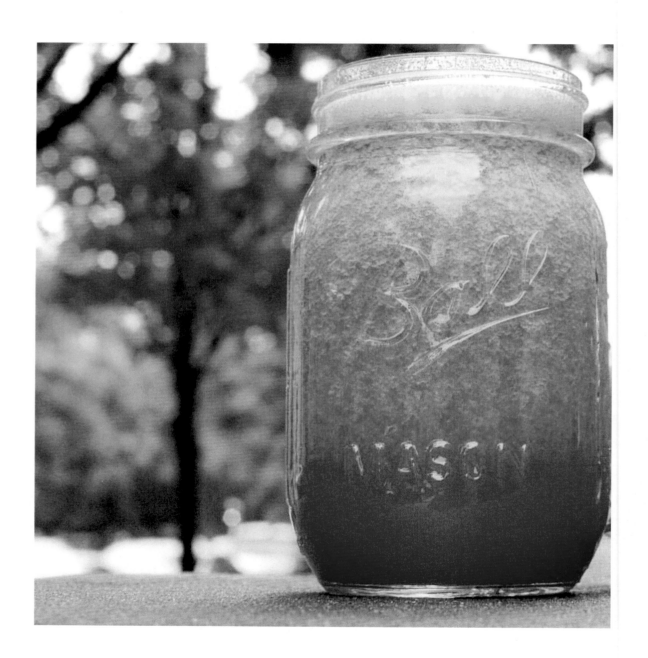

The combination of raw food, juicing, enzymes, and colonics have been extremely successful at resolving all kinds of chronic and systemic illnesses at places like Hippocrates in Florida. If I had a little time and money, it would be worth it to go there and reset your body post-chemo or radiation or in the early stages of cancer.

I should add that I had acupuncture and a massage three times a week for two months while on this program. I did not eat wheat, sugar, dairy, or other animal products—except maybe at a birthday party, a few bites here and there. I drank three liters of purified water daily. Every two weeks, I went to an energy healer like Penney Leyshon. I also went to a Brennan therapist, a hypnotist, and a craniosacral practitioner. I exercised almost every day, swimming laps and/or Pilates or yoga.

In the past four years, since the cancer and the tumor disappeared and the scars healed themselves, I have slacked off in terms of supplements—and I have to admit, I don't look nearly as good!

I do currently take Essiac tea every morning as a prophylactic and have been for the past three months, with no adverse effects.

The above regimen cost me more than $1,500 a month, and that doesn't even include the doctors and there was only so long I could afford it.

But this is what worked for me.

Remember, this is an arsenal. It is a group effort. Diet, acupuncture, supplements, exercise, energy work, prayer or meditation, therapy, getting A LOT of rest.

In terms of energy work, it all sounds very woo-woo, but there is a growing body of evidence showing that it makes a pronounced difference in speeding healing, shrinking tumors and reducing pain. So experiment with whatever you can find—there's a lot out there. Just remember to say NO, very firmly, if anyone makes you feel uncomfortable.

It's not enough to do one or two things because cancer is a big disease. And it's here to teach you something. So do everything you can to learn the lesson and move on.

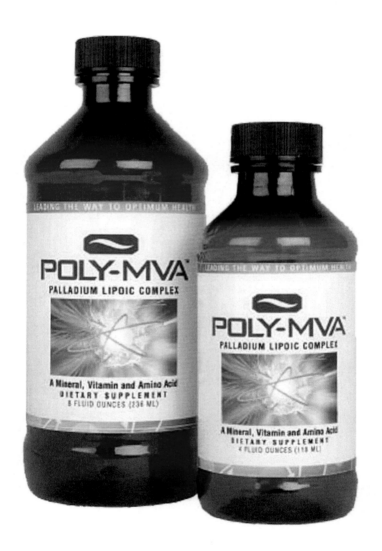

My #1 Supplement

PolyMVA gives you the energy
to survive chemotherapy.

CHAPTER EIGHT: My #1 Supplement

One of the supplements I always recommend to anyone I know who has cancer is PolyMVA. It's both effective with chemotherapy and/or radiation or on its own. I also use it as system boost any time I feel anything coming on, it supports multiple body systems. In my case, I started taking it while I was getting chemo, along with CoQ10. I noticed that, despite being around young kids and spending lots of time in public places, I didn't catch so much as a cold. On the one day when I started to get sniffly, I took an extra dose of the PolyMVA (normally, I took two teaspoons in a glass of water, three or four times a day) then two hours' later, a big dose of vitamin c and the next day it was gone. I was also incredibly resilient, I was able to take Pilates during chemo and start swimming laps again within two weeks of stopping.

PolyMVA is a dark liquid combination of thiamin, the mineral palladium and alpha lipoic acid (poly) along with other minerals, vitamins, and amino acids (MVA). To me, it tastes—probably because of all the B-vitamins—like marmite without any salt. Bad, but not gag-worthy. Clearly, the clever name was not created by a copywriter. Unlike a lot of supplemental combinations, it has been subject to 20 years of clinical research and four FDA reviews.

There are scores of long-term survivors who strongly believe in the product and share stories in person, online and in podcasts. A man called Walter Davis actually has created a regular PolyMVA radio show in which he invites people to share their experience and give their testimonials.

I was lucky enough to interview Gary Matson, a retired pastor, who works for PolyMVA and coordinates with the doctors and their protocols. He had actually been a bereavement counselor when his 62-year-old wife was diagnosed with stage-4 brain cancer. His son was a doctor in Southern California and got them the best allopathic medical care. They'd followed every traditional protocol but, finally, were told she had two weeks to live. In hospice, he learned about PolyMVA and he started giving it to his wife. He and the family were astonished that her health began improving and within three months, an MRI showed that all of her tumors had stopped growing. She became her cheerful self again and her family was thrilled to have her back. Within five months, all of her previous tumors were gone. (Unfortunately, she passed when a different tumor reached the brain stem but the 6-month reprieve was priceless to her family). Gary learned later in talking

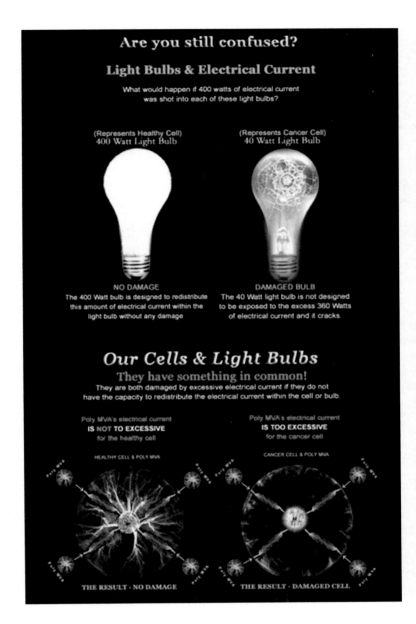

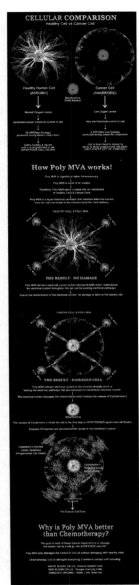

with the metabolic cardiologist, Stephen Sinatra, that the brain stem has poor blood flow and absorption and CoQ10 could have potentiated the absorption of the Poly-MVA. Now every cancer client is encouraged to include CoQ10 and there are a number of brain stem tumor survivors.

Matson explained that many people don't realize that for cancer patients and their families what does not get measured by is Quality of Life: those last months were precious. Their PolyMVA experience added 6 months' of life to enjoy and spend with their loved one.

PolyMVA was discovered by a scientist, researcher and originally, a dentist, from Long Island, NY named Merrill Garnett. His experience in oral cancers and his exposure in chemistry opened the door for him to ponder, develop and eventually create Poly-MVA from a new understanding of nutrition and cellular metabolism and energetics, the Warburg effect. He worked initially at the Stony Brook incubator labs in Long Island. He eventually realized that a complex of high-level, high-powered ingredients like B1, B2, B12, rhodium, palladium, and alpha-lipoic acid were crucial. The design allowed it to cross into the brain through the blood brain barrier. The combination of ingredients is water and fat-soluble and therefore available to all cells. It protects normal cells and supports their mitochondria by increasing energy through the electron transport chain, allowing the cells to function properly. These nutrients support the body in repairing the cancer cells and improving the quality of all the normal surrounding cells.

I'm not a biochemist myself so my explanations are not as clear as the infographics. The end result is that the PolyMVA works by "flooding" all cells, even the anaerobic cancer cells with energy and increasing their oxygen pathways, thus turning on the mechanism or pathway of normal cell death or "short circuiting or electrocuting" them, while increasing the energy and strengthening the normal cells to keep them operating normally and not from mutating into cancer.

According to the doctors and current research, the transformation of the cancer takes time—cancer both develops and fades away slowly. That's why it takes three to six months on "loading doses." In natural medicine, this means a larger beginning dose that sets the healing process in motion. A loading dose can be six to twelve teaspoons a day. I was taking eight—or one teaspoon for every 10 to 15 pounds of body weight. While nothing has an instant effect on one's sonograms/scans, within a week or two of this dose, almost every cancer patient has a marked increase in energy and appetite and color back in their cheeks, what they call the QOL.

In about four months, most people begin stabilizing and many times the body starts shrinking the tumors.

Because it's a liquid, it's very easily absorbed into the bloodstream even if the digestive system is compromised. Some doctors even use it intravenously for patients.

The main disadvantage with any non-traditional approaches is the out-of-pocket cost. The mineral palladium is expensive, so PolyMVA costs $180 for a large 8oz. bottle—which is even more than it cost when I was taking it. In my case, that meant about $500 a month.

PolyMVA is not a typical supplement in cost or action and probably won't get cheaper. On the other hand, I was happy to see that Iron Man used palladium in his arc reactor to get his power (though it was poisoning him, until he learned how to stabilize it, which is what Dr. Garnett did, sequestering/hiding the mineral or energy source inside the Alpha Lipoic Acid and Thiamin).

Taking coQ10—and I recommend epic4health as one of the best distributors of the product—increases the bioavailability of the PolyMVA but adds to the cost. Also, in order to make it most effective, it's crucial that you change your diet and your lifestyle, like giving up sugar and processed foods—which a lot of people find extremely difficult to do, even when faced with death as an alternative.

Along with other high-dose protocols, you want to time the dosages and treatments so that you do not interfere with another product. For example, vitamin C can minimize the poly support, so I waited 2 hours between doses.

The advantage, if you're on the East Coast or Europe, is that you can call the customer service at Amarc Enterprises (the Manufacturer) until quite late since they are in California. My personal contact was a woman called Vivien Ariola. They give you friendly advice on how to take it and/or modify your diet. Some of them are cancer survivors themselves.

Today, there are a number of doctors who have experimented with or prescribe PolyMVA for their patients. Amongst them, the late cardiologist, Dr. Rudy Falk and oncologist James Forsythe. Forsythe has used and studied PolyMVA in an outcome-based study since 2004 in over 1700 patients. The success rates for the PolyMVA combination are as high as 60% remission. Another metabolic cardiologist, Stephen Sinatra, recommends it for many other health conditions simply because so many conditions start with oxidative stress and metabolic dysfunction.

Personally, I found that my oncologist at Memorial Sloan Kettering was not averse to this supplement. On the other hand, I was such a squeaky wheel that she may have just hoped I would continue getting treatment.

In your search for integrative, alternative or complementary cancer medicines, it's good to know which ones are not scams or weird "healing secrets." These days, I seem to get an email or two a day with those subject lines: "The cures your doctors don't want you to know!" or "Secret healing from the Bible," or "Weird spice CURES cancer."

Basically, either they don't really explain what they are or they are simply overpriced combinations of garlic and turmeric, which you are better off buying from a reputable supplement company.

Since I get zero benefit from any of my recommendations, and I've tested it on myself and friends, you can trust your intuition here. I'd recommend that everyone who has cellular, metabolic dysfunction or cancer—especially leukemia, bone and/or brain cancer, or even, heart disease—add PolyMVA to their healing arsenal.

Remember, you will be healed. Keep repeating to yourself—

I am healed,
I am healthy,
I am vibrant,
I am cancer-free.

Essiac Tea

Herbal healing.
Native American herbs to know.

CHAPTER NINE: The Herbal Cure. Essiac Tea.

Since I've recovered, people often call or email me to talk a friend or family member who has just discovered he/she has cancer of one kind or another.

I tell them my story and give them tips about what they can do to heal naturally, as well as what they might do in conjunction with chemo. I've been impressed that people who take the information and run with it have incredible results. Cancer recedes, diabetes disappears, aggressive tumors turn benign. Even if it is a few years since their cancer was treated, changing their diets, breathing, exercising, and taking supplements has changed their lives. They are energetic and vibrant, their skin glows, they are optimistic and active.

Usually, almost everyone I talk to gets really excited about the options available to them. With a little research, there are so many ways to heal cancer these days—and heal it in a way that overhauls your life for the better—that people come away feeling relieved and positive about the challenge.

Unfortunately, three-quarters of the people I advise then go to the hospital and get frightened. Their doctors say things like, "Well, if you take these supplements, we can't help you..."

Or, as they said to a friend, "If you want to risk your life like that, go ahead, because we can't guarantee the results of alternative treatment."

So remember: Healing cancer, even more than almost any other disease, IS possible—but it's uncertain, no matter which method. All of our bodies are different and react differently. All of our minds and souls have different lessons to learn. Whether you choose the traditional route or the naturopathic one or a combination, *THERE IS NO GUARANTEE.* Just because the doctor/healer says they have success with one method or another, doesn't mean it will work on you.

For instance, if you have a virus and a doctor mistakenly prescribes you antibiotics and you get even sicker and end up in the hospital, you don't get anything back from the doctor. There is no money-back guarantee on healing. And worse, there is no health-back guarantee. This is even scarier when you are dealing with your kids.

So here's the other thing, YOU live in your body. You know it better than anyone else and you have for years. See what you feel comfortable with. Try one thing and see if it makes you feel better. There is nothing wrong with testing the experiences and listening to your body.

If it's your kid—remember, this child lived IN your body—you were there from his/her earliest moments. No one knows your child better than you do.

My recommendation: Cancer is systemic, so never stick to any single therapy. You need to heal mind, body, and soul. If it makes you feel better to follow an oncologist's orders, do that. But also try the dietary changes and supplements. Try hypnotherapy, try polarity, try Brennan healing. Try acupuncture, infrared heat, and vitamin therapy. Try intravenous glutathione, meditation, and Chinese medicine. See what makes you feel like you are healing.

Recently, I discovered **Essaic tea**.

It's a brewed herbal mixture that was created by a Native American tribe called the Ojibwa that uses local plant roots, bark and leaves to kill cancer and also normalize diabetes and HIV. It started being used in mainstream healing by a nurse called Rene Caisse in Canada. She had such success with using it to heal bottom-the-barrel cancer cases that it exploded.

Since I've been studying herbal medicine and Chinese medicine, I cross-referenced the four main ingredients with my textbooks and what I've learned. I also put in hours with my biology textbooks and reading testimonials and research online.

I should add that Essiac Tea has a tumultuous history with the mainstream—and even slightly alternative—medical establishment. Andrew Weil, for instance, says you should avoid it. But he also says that the formula was never passed on correctly by Rene Caisse. Apparently, Caisse refused to divulge her ingredients to the drug companies because she believed the product should be cheap and free and readily available. She did give it to Memorial Sloan Kettering and, interestingly, there are studies on their websites regarding certain ingredients, but from what I've read, she got angry at the way they handled it (they froze the herbs, making them much weaker) and took it all back.

That said, there are so many good testimonials—most people have bought a jar of vitamins on Amazon with fewer good reviews. And you can buy it on Amazon as capsules, pre-made liquid, and dried herbs. It is also sold under the name Flor-Essence with the addition of kelp (good for the thyroid), red clover (builds iron and strength), watercress (purifies the blood, tones the kidneys and reduces inflammation), and blessed thistle (strengthens and tones the liver).

The ingredients are as follows:

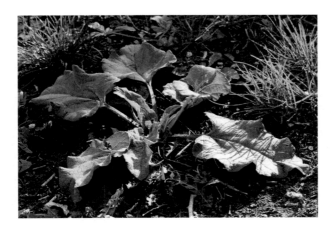

Burdock Root — which has been used for centuries in Chinese medicine to address a multitude of illnesses, amongst them diabetes, gout, wrinkles (aging skin), measles, and hypoglycemia. It has anti-tumor effects and is used in India and Russia in cancer treatments. It's also been used to cure fibroids. Burdock root is the main ingredient in Essaic tea. It's a pretty common weed that grows along roadsides in the U.S. and Canada.

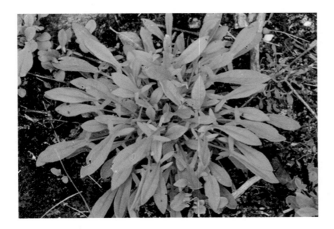

Sheep Sorrell — this grows wild all over North America, in fields and meadows. It's an astringent and a diuretic with a tangy, lemony taste. Traditionally, it's been used to treat fevers, scurvy, and diarrhea, but it's also nice as a salad green. In Essaic tea, it's an anti-tumor agent, as well as an anti-bacterial. Kids like to chew on it, calling it sour grass. It should be taken in small quantities—and its proportions are quite small in the Essaic mixture.

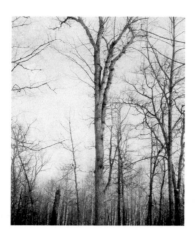

Slippery Elm — you might recognize this name from natural sore throat and cough remedies. It coats the throat, esophagus, and even bowels when ingested, which makes it great for mitigating the effects of chemo and/or radiation on your mucus membranes. When applied topically, it calms and soothes irritation on the skin as well. While, according to Memorial Sloan Kettering, it doesn't have anti-tumor effects, it does have antioxidant and anti-inflammatory qualities. Its mucillagenous (slippery, right?) qualities make it especially good for coating the stomach in IBS. People even eat it as a highly-digestible food. The trees grow in the Northern U.S. and Canada.

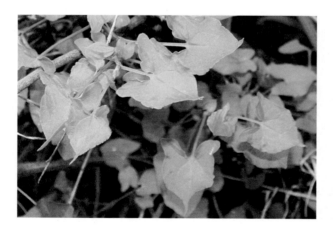

Turkey or Indian Rhubarb — this plant has been used in herbal remedies for over 2,000 years. It has both anti-inflammatory and anti-oxidant effects. In Essaic tea, it's used for its anthroquinones, emodin, and rhein, which have tumor killing capacities. Anthroquinones are also good for strengthening the lungs, especially after chemotherapy or radiation. Finally, it's said that the tea can be used for controlling menopausal symptoms like hot flashes.

It seems incredible. If you have any health issues that affect the pancreas or liver, from diabetes to hepatitis to HIV or cancer, you might try this tea. Some people, like Flor-Essence, add additional herbs but these are the four main ones.

(The tedious part is making the tea. This isn't the kind where you buy a teabag and put it in a cup with hot water. It is actually a herbal extract or tincture, so it is boiled for quite a long time, then strained and reduced again. Then you have to sterilize and fill a bottle with the thick, dark substance and keep it in the fridge. The advantage is that it lasts for several weeks that way and you only take a tiny amount in the morning and the evening, ideally on an empty stomach.)

Think about it this way, if you have a horrible sinus infection and you go to the doctor for antibiotics, you are probably still going to drink soup and grapefruit juice, take vitamin C, and maybe a hot toddy and/or watch some funny movies on Netflix.

The doctor will tell you that all these other things won't make any difference. But, if you really want to get well fast, you'll decide that you want to put in the extra effort.

Along with meditating and speaking gently to your body and your cancer, it's worth it to use every piece of soul and body strengthening weapons reinforcements in your arsenal.

Just know that if you want to be well, listen to your body. Love it. Put in the time to treat yourself with love and respect. Who knows what miracles you could make happen?

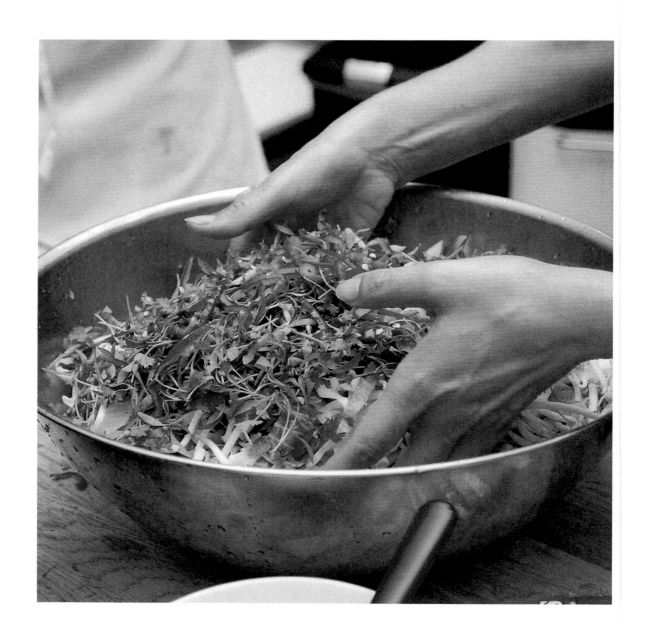

CHAPTER TEN

What's Left To Eat?
Eating to Heal.

Recipes for an AntiCancer Diet.

CHAPTER TEN: What's Left To Eat? Eating To Heal.

At this this point, you've read all the things I gave up—all the allergens (wheat, dairy, soy, peanuts), processed foods, preservatives, sugar, animal products (except for a little bit of organic, grass-fed meat or chicken or wild fish). When the weather was warm, I ate totally raw—and gave up the rest of the grains, too. You might be despairing—what IS there to eat?

As it turns out, I did not have to become a breatharian. This gentle, detox diet would probably do wonders for almost anyone. It's very good for soothing the body, as well as giving it the support it needs to heal itself if you are trying to kickstart a weight loss program, lower your blood pressure or cholesterol, or simply soothe your body during a stressful time

A lot of people follow the ketogenic diet very successfully to "starve" their cancer out. In my case, I didn't do that. Instead, I tried to make my diet at least 80% vegetables. These days, if you live in a major metropolitan area, you'll find many of the ingredients and even pre-prepared food in health food stores, supermarkets, and on Amazon.com. Any time I mention vegetables here, I mean organic and non-GMO—you must read labels carefully. If you absolutely can't find organic, wash and peel the vegetables before you use them. But personally, I think anyone with cancer should not eat ANY pesticides or GMO products, so it may be better to bite the bullet and try to find organic or at least, locally-grown from small farms.

Dr. Mercola's website is also great resource for news on natural health and cancer-fighting diet strategies.

I put my diet together by reading cancer diets online and by consulting with nutritionist Joel Fuhrman, so some of my recipes are modified from his book which is totally worth reading when you are feeling strong.

Any time I use salt I use himalayan pink salt, but you can also use sea salt. Commercial table salt is bleached and refined and, according to Max Gerson, the doctor who created Gerson therapy, it causes an imbalance in the body.

A few suggestions: Try to make everything as fresh as possible, don't eat leftovers too often and **NEVER MICROWAVE** anything. Microwaving heats food by making the water molecules speed up and there is a theory that that affects the chemical composition of the food and how it reacts with the water in your body. Remember you are 70% water.

A ban on microwaving can be tough in the morning when one is in a rush. If I really don't have time, I eat a handful of raw nuts along with a dried or fresh fig or two—as long as it doesn't have any preservatives or sugar. I tend not to have smoothies for breakfast even though they're fast, but for me, they are too intense in the morning.

BEFORE BREAKFAST

Here's what I do in the morning: I have two tablespoons of Essiac tea and then a big glass of water with two spoonfuls of PolyMVA. Then I do some oil pulling since chemo can do a lot of damage to your gums and teeth. Lots of dentists don't like to work on cancer patients as we get infections so easily.

For my oil pulling, I use one tablespoon of raw coconut or sesame oil and sometimes, one drop of myrhh or thieves essential oils because they are a good antibacterial. I put it in my mouth and swirl and swish it around while I take a shower and walk the dog or read emails for five to 20 minutes. I spit it into a paper towel or directly into the garbage and go rinse my mouth and/or brush my teeth.

Next I have a **green juice**:

- 4 or 5 leaves of lacinato kale or 2 or 3 of regular kale
- A small bunch of cilantro or parsley
- A small bunch of dandelion greens, collard greens, mustard greens, and/or swiss chard
- Broccoli stems or any raw vegetable parts that you didn't cook
- 1 small lemon
- 1 to 1 1/2 of a cucumber, depending on the size
- 4 stalks of celery
- 1 1/2 inch of fresh ginger
- 1/4 to 1/2 of a tart green apple, to taste

All the ingredients must be organic (except maybe the ginger because it's hard to find), because when you drink the juice, you are getting a super concentrated dose of the vegetable and you don't want a concentrated dose of pesticides with it. I put all these in my Omega VRT 350 juicer.

I mix up the combinations so it doesn't get boring. Sometimes I add a couple of carrots instead of apples. I don't add beets because they don't agree with me but they are good for the blood. You can add some from time to time, but not too much because, of course, they are so sugary.

If I am in a hurry, I buy a cold-pressed Mother Earth from the **Juice Press** or the Detoxifier from **Juice Generation**. Or the Squeeze truck's Stand and Deliver. All three brands were great because they didn't use hpp—a way of preserving the juice by squeezing all the air out of it (which tragically kills some of the enzymes) and means that it really isn't raw any more.

Either before or after, I drink a cup of hot water with a big squeeze of fresh lemon juice. I also take my probiotics.

I then drink green or black tea (with almond or hemp milk) and take a tablespoon of coconut oil or an MCT oil to feed my brain and slow down the absorption of the caffeine.

In Paul Pitchford's famous *Healing with Whole Foods*, he suggests waiting for an hour or two after you wake up before you have solid foods. This is a brilliant book on healing the body with food but it's heavy reading so if you are in the throes of chemo or radiation, maybe a friend can start it out for you.

After the juice, tea, coconut oil, and everything else, you probably won't be hungry for a little while. When you are ready, here are some possible foods.

FOR BREAKFAST:

Chia Porridge:

- 2 tablespoons of chia seeds
- 2 tablespoons of shelled hemp seeds
- 2 tablespoons of flax seeds
- 1 handful of goji berries (for sweetness)
- Pinch of salt

I put everything together in a bowl and then add a cup of almond or coconut milk, stir it up well and let it sit. Within a few minutes, it will be thick and custardy. If it's too thick, I add more nut milk and/or a little hot water to warm it up. Sometimes, if I really need it a little sweeter, I add a sprinkle of coconut sugar on the top. You could also use a few drops of stevia extract but I don't like the aftertaste. You'll notice that if you don't mix it in, it hits your tongue first and you need less.

Black Rice Toast and Avocado:

Toast a slice of Food for Life Black Rice bread (which tastes more like a soft-baked cracker than bread, it's relatively low-carb and gluten-free), top it with artichoke pesto (see below) and slices of fresh avocado. If want extra protein, I might add an organic, cage-free scrambled egg or a strip of organic turkey bacon or some chopped roasted almonds.

Artichoke Pesto:

I put this on everything—from quinoa pasta to grilled salmon. You can buy it but it's better if you make it because there are theories that corn and canola oil contribute to the growth of tumors whereas olive, flax, and coconut oil do not. So here's a recipe, but I suggest you play around with the ingredients to taste. I don't use parmesan cheese but if you do, make sure it is organic and adjust the salt accordingly.

- Small bunch (1/4 to 1/2 cup chopped) cilantro/coriander
- 8 garlic cloves
- 4 tablespoons of lemon juice
- 1/2 teaspoon of cayenne (or maybe a fresh green chili if you like it spicy)
- 1 cup of walnuts (especially good for prostate cancer)
- 1 cup of olive oil
- 1, 8 oz package of frozen artichokes, thawed and chopped
- Sea salt to taste

I just put it all in the Vitamix and pulse until it is a chunky but spreadable texture. It keeps for a week or two in the refrigerator. You can dip carrot sticks in it or mix in more olive oil and lemon and use it as salad dressing. Artichokes are great for clearing the liver and blood.

Oatmeal:

Joel Fuhrman suggested I make it using steel-cut oats which are quite slow-cooking. I used to cook a large amount in advance and then put it in a container in my fridge and heat it up a little at a time.

- 2 cups of oatmeal
- 3 cups of water
- 1 cup of fresh apple cider
- 1 tablespoon of organic blackstrap molasses
- Cinnamon, cloves, cardamom, nutmeg, nigella sativa (onion seed), and ginger
- 1/4 teaspoon of salt
- 1/2 cup of chopped almonds, hazelnuts and/or walnuts cup of chopped dried figs which (along with sour apples) are one of the fruits that good for killing cancer cells.

I eat the oatmeal as is or I add a little nut milk to make it more liquidy. If you desperately need it sweeter, add a tiny bit of raw honey on top after you serve yourself. In Chinese medicine, all the spices are warming and cancer quite often makes a person cold, so this is a Qi-building tonic.

Indian Scrambled Eggs:

- 3 scallions
- 1 to 2 cloves of garlic, chopped
- 1/2 cup chopped coriander
- 1/2 teaspoon of fresh ginger, chopped very fine
- 1/4 teaspoon turmeric powder
- 1 green chili (with the seeds removed if you don't want it too spicy, wear gloves or ask for help while doing this as your skin is very sensitive during chemo)
- 1 or 2 free range eggs
- 2 tablespoons of coconut oil (or grass-fed butter)

Heat the oil or butter in the pan and lightly brown the garlic, scallions, and ginger, add a bit of sea salt or himalayan pink salt. Then add the eggs, the coriander and the chilies and cook quickly so the eggs are still slightly soft and the coriander bright green. Eat it up!

You can, of course, just make ordinary scrambled eggs. This is just to jazz it up. Also, while I was having chemo, I found myself craving strong sharp tastes to awaken my appetite. I was tired and not very hungry most of the time. Since I refused to take prednisone (or steroids) with my chemo, I kept my bones strong but I had bad nausea. I counteracted the nausea with A LOT Of fresh ginger. It actually worked very well.

Sometimes, I have a small amount of grilled salmon over baby kale with artichoke pesto and olive oil on top.

If I'm in a rush but want something savory, I chop some broccoli, quickly parboil it in the tiniest bit of water, and eat it with tamari or a little bit of miso.

For Lunch:

Smoothie:

I usually save my smoothies for lunch because they keep me full for a long time. My favorite smoothie is still the same:

- 1 avocado
- 3 to 4 leaves of kale or swiss chard, stems removed
- Packet of unsweetened acai
- 1 scoop of delgado protocol stem cell strong (this has lots of good mushrooms and parasite-killing herbs) but you can use other brands.
- 1 cup of vanilla hemp or macadamia nut milk
- 1 cup or so of coconut water, more if it gets too thick

Big Green Salad:

I am very flexible and organic (not the certified kind) when I cook and even more so with salad because I think respecting your vegetables and their combinations is key, otherwise chewing it feels like a chore for horses. I do what the French do and start with a big salad bowl. I make the dressing at the bottom, put the salad on top and then toss it all together. All the measurements are approximate and you will have to see what works for you.

- 1/4 to 1/2 cup of extra virgin organic, cold-pressed olive oil
- 2 to 3 big tablespoons of pesto, basil, or artichoke, or one of each.
- 1 tsp black olive tapenade (check the ingredients to make sure there are no preservatives)
- A few anchovies very finely chopped (optional)
- 1/4 cup of fresh herbs—whatever you have, basil, coriander, oregano... if you use thyme or rosemary, of course, you will need much less and have to chop very finely
- A few squeezes of fresh lemon

Stir this all up and taste, maybe add some Coconut Aminos if it needs more salt.

If it's summer, you can chop in some fresh tomatoes, but otherwise, don't eat unripe tomatoes. In Chinese medicine, nightshades cause inflammation and unripe tomatoes seem especially suspect.

Add a small washed bag of organic baby greens (spinach, arugula, kale, swiss chard, watercress, whatever you can find). If I have some leftovers in the fridge—like roast chicken or grilled fish or meat or vegetables—I heat them a little in a hot oven (just in case of mold or bacteria) and throw them in, too. You can also add cooked beans, edamame, or corn (as long as it is organic and not canned or frozen).

If you want to add something really tough and chewy, like carrots or cabbage, be sure and grate it well first so that it mixes together with everything else. After it's tossed, throw in the broccoli or kale sprouts because they wilt very quickly—though peat shoots really hold their own. Eat this up immediately, it won't keep.

Vegetable Slaw:

I make this more like an Asian-style slaw and it's good way to eat lots of cabbage and carrots. If you add cucumber, know that it will get much more drippy and liquid. You can do that whole thing of removing the seeds of the cucumbers first but it's tedious.

- 1/4 head of cabbage chopped
- 3 or 4 carrots grated
- 1 daikon grated (daikon is a japanese radish that has cancer-killing properties)
- 1 cup of mung bean sprouts
- 1/2 cup of broccoli or kale sprouts
- 1 cucumber grated (optional)

- 1/2 cup of broccoli or kale sprouts
- 1 cucumber grated (optional)
- 1/4 cup chopped almonds or hazelnuts (I use these instead because peanuts cause inflammation and when you have cancer, you are trying to keep your body as calm and cool as you can)
- 1/4 to 1/2 cup fresh basil, coriander and mint, chopped

In a small bowl, mix the sauce:

- 1 clove garlic minced
- 1 small shallot or three scallions, chopped
- 1/2 teaspoon minced ginger
- 1 teaspoon nam pla (fish sauce—more to taste)
- 1/2 teaspoon raw honey
- Juice of 1 lime or lemon
- 1 to 4 thai chili (seeds removed) chopped very fine, depending on how spicy you want it

Toss it all veggies together and then add the sauce a little at time to taste. You can put it all in fridge to marinate for a day if you like. If you do prepare it ahead of time, don't add the cucumbers or sprouts 'til you're just about to eat. This makes me one serving, but I eat a lot of salad.

The dressing is very Asian-inspired, but you can try out your favorites. If you decide you want to use a mayonnaise-type dressing for a classic cole slaw, I'd suggest you make your own. Most commercial mayonnaises use soybean oil which is usually GMO, pesticide-laced, and too high in omega-6s. If you can find a local, small batch organic mayonnaise using olive oil and cage-free eggs, go for it. I just found out that I am highly sensitive to eggs and soy so that's another reason I don't use mayonnaise or vegannaise.

Zucchini "Pasta" with Basil Pesto:

For this, you need a spiralizer. They are not too expensive and they are a super cool kitchen tool to have around because you can cut spirals of all kinds of vegetables and that makes them more interesting to eat.

- 1 to 2 small zucchinis/courgettes
- 2 to 3 tablespoons of vegan basil pesto (this just means pesto that has no cheese, but you can just as easily do it with a little parmesan)

This is kind of a trick food because it's so easy. You chop off the top, impale the zucchini in the spiralizer, and put a bowl in front of it. Then spin it around until long, "spaghetti" strands start filling up your bowl. Toss it with the pesto and add more or less to taste. It's wonderful to eat if you are missing the "pasta" texture. You have to eat this relatively quickly too, as the zucchini can get watery from the salt.

For Snacks:

I usually have lots of fresh carrots, celery, daikon, jicama, and cucumber chopped up that I can dip into hummus, artichoke pesto, or even olive oil and lemon.

I like oat cakes (homemade made using coconut oil or grass-fed raw butter rather than goosefat or Nairn's) with almond, hazelnut, or cashew butter.

I also eat Brad's Nasty Hot Kale Chips. You can see that spicy food is a theme for me. There are other versions, too. But it's good way to keep up your cruciferous vegetables. If you can't buy them and you don't have a dehydrator, I suggest tossing kale with salt and garlic and putting it in the oven at the lowest temperature you can possibly use and letting it dry out for a couple of hours. Just check it from time to time to make sure they are not burning up.

Tart green apples or fresh or dried figs are the few fruits that you can eat without much trouble. I wouldn't eat large quantities but they are a nice snack when you need sweets.

Hazelnuts, pumpkin seeds, sunflower seeds, and chickpeas all have anti-cancer properties, so you can eat a handful of them whenever you want. These days you can buy them in all different flavors, too.

I just discovered this recipe online for when you are craving chocolate.

Coconut Chocolate Sea Salt Fudge:

Melt an equal amount of coconut oil and unsweetened chocolate into a pan at very low heat so the fat doesn't separate from the cocoa solids, add a pinch of himalayan or sea salt.

Sweeten with stevia extract or (lo han guo) monk fruit—two low-glycemic sweeteners that you can actually eat from time to time. Don't add too much though because they can still trigger sugar cravings if it gets too sweet.

Ladle mixture carefully into an ice cube tray.

Put in freezer for thirty minutes.

When solid, loosen from ice cube tray with a knife and pop out into a plate or freezer-safe container. Return to freezer 'til you are ready to eat.

You can eat one or two when your sweet cravings are driving you crazy.

One of the best way to detox from your sugar cravings is a glass of water with a tablespoon of Bragg's Apple Cider vinegar. Put all the sweets out of sight and then chew some chlorella tablets which are also good for quelling sugar and junk food cravings.

For Dinner:

If it is winter, I like a hot, hearty meal to warm me up—and also heat up my kitchen—in the evening. But there are sometimes, especially in the summer, when I find I don't feel very hungry at dinner and I skip it all together. For the most part, if you have cancer, I don't believe you should force yourself to eat if you are not hungry. It's better to rest and eat small amounts of food when you do feel hungry. It may seem scary when you lose weight, but rest assured it will come back when your body is in balance. **DO NOT EAT JUNK FOOD IN AN ATTEMPT TO GAIN WEIGHT!** That can backfire and weaken your immune system even more.

In fact, there are some studies showing that fasting during chemotherapy actually kills cancer cells faster.

Here a bunch of warm things you can make so you eat more vegetables without feeling like you are eating a tragic meal of cold leaves while everyone else has something hearty.

Lentil or Split Pea Soup:

If I making dinner for myself (without kids), I usually make soup. Since I am an Asian, I like the taste of browned onions and garlic, so I'll start by browning them in a little coconut or olive oil.

- 1 onion, sliced or chopped
- 2 to 3 cloves of garlic, minced or sliced
- 2 to 3 tablespoons of olive or coconut oil
- 1 cup of dried lentils, split peas or dried beans—or a combination. If you are impatient like me, I suggest you soak them the night before, or in the morning when you are doing your oil-pulling.
- 2 carrots, chopped
- 2 stalks of celery chopped
- 1/2 to 1 cup of maitake, shitake, and reishi mushrooms, chopped
- Any other vegetables, cooked or raw, you have lying around (broccoli, kale, cabbage, sweet potatoes, chop them up and throw them in)
- 4 cups of purified water

Brown the onions and garlic with a little salt in the oil. You can even add the other raw vegetables and brown them a little because it changes their texture and adds a little sweetness, but you don't have to. Then add the beans/peas/lentils, mushrooms, and water and anything else you want to put in. I often add anything that is leftover in the fridge— sometimes it's a little roast chicken or steak or fish, sometimes it's raw or roasted vegetables. Then you let it simmer forever (that's what it seems like to me) but it can be a few hours unless it's well-soaked. You have to check on it and add water when the pulses suck it up, so that it doesn't get too thick. Once it's finished, you can eat it immediately and save some for the next day or two as well.

Roasted Broccoli:

This is a delicious way to prepare broccoli that my youngest daughter discovered online and that we have customized. We make it often because everyone likes to eat it and we go through several heads of broccoli in one sitting.

- 1 head of broccoli
- 4 to 5 tablespoons of olive oil
- 3 cloves of minced garlic
- Sea salt/himalayan salt to taste
- Freshly-ground black pepper (only because it tastes better)
- 1 fresh lemon to squeeze

Preheat the oven to 425 (Farenheit). Cut up the head of broccoli, separating the florets and leaving the stems (you can juice those tomorrow morning). Put it in a bowl and toss with the olive oil and garlic. Sprinkle with salt and pepper to taste. Spread the broccoli on a cookie sheet. Put it in the oven at 425 for about 15 minutes, check on it from time to time. If it's nicely browned around the edges and slightly crispy, you can take it out. If it feels too soggy, reduce the heat to 300 and leave it in for a few minutes longer so that it gets drier and crisper.

Put it in a serving dish and squeeze a little lemon over it if you like. Or don't, if you don't feel like it.

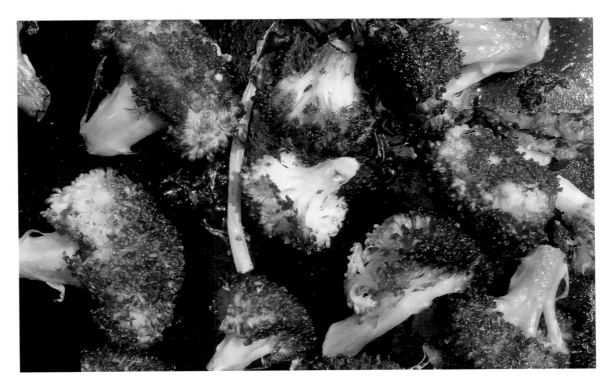

Roasted Brussels Sprouts:

This is similar to the broccoli, though sometimes bitter Brussel sprouts become slightly sweet and crispy and quite luscious after roasting—but they burn much more quickly than broccoli, so keep your eye on them.

- 2 containers of Brussel sprouts, maybe a pound and a half
- 3 cloves of garlic
- 3 tablespoons of coconut oil or grass-fed butter
- 1/2 cup chopped hazelnuts
- Himalayan or sea salt to taste

Preheat the oven to 400. Rinse the sprouts, remove the outer leaves, chop them in quarters, and put them in a big bowl. Toss them with the oil or butter and garlic. Put them on a cookie sheet or a wide baking pan. Roast for 10 minutes, then toss in the hazelnuts and reduce the heat to 300. Roast for another five to 10 minutes, until nicely browned but not burned.

Roasted Sweet Potatoes or Yams:

This is a regular dish in my house and the prep is quite similar to the other roasted things.

- 4 big yams, washed and chopped into bite-size pieces
- 4 or 5 shallots, peeled, maybe cut in half if they are big
- 1 or 2 additional root vegetables if you have some, washed and chopped
- 8 to 10 big cloves of garlic
- Vietnamese cinnamon, ground
- Fine herbes or Trader Joe's 21 Salute
- Sea salt or Himalayan salt
- 4 tablespoons of coconut oil

Preheat the oven to 450. Basically, add the vegetables (and shallots and garlic) to a roasting pan. I use my 13 x 9 cake pan. Sprinkle with spices, salt, and coconut oil and stir it all up with a big wooden spoon. Shake the pan slightly so everything is distributed evenly and put it in the oven. I leave them there for about 20 minutes and then I reduce the heat to 350 and leave them in there for a really long time—like maybe another 45 minutes. If I have time, I take them out in the middle and toss them around the pan a bit so they cook evenly. But even if I don't, they seem to do fine, the slightly burned ones taste nice too.

Sautéed Kale or Spinach:

I go back and forth between the two—sautéed kale has a lot more body and can stand up to longer cooking so it can become a nice combination of bitter and sweet. Sautéed spinach becomes soft and soothing and it's a good comfort food.

If I am making sautéed spinach, I heat a few tablespoons of olive oil first along with slices of three or four garlic cloves and a few sprinkles of himalayan or sea salt and pepper. I like to let the sliced garlic brown a little before I add a big bunch of spinach. I add salt to taste and cook the spinach just until it's wilted and bright green.

If I am sautéing kale, I add the oil and garlic but then I de-vein (take out the hard stems) and chop the bunch of kale finely and add it as soon as I am finished chopping it. I cook it for quite a long time so it is not too chewy.

What is crucial is that you never heat the olive oil to smoking point. Olive oil is full of anti-oxidants as long as it is not overheated. So let it brown your garlic gently. If you feel you want a nice crispy, stir-fry sensibility, switch to coconut oil or macadamia nut oil which is better at high heat.

Tandoori Roasted Cauliflower:

I adapted this from a recipe I found on PureWow—and you could use theirs instead, just never use "vegetable" oil—always choose coconut, olive, or palm fruit – as corn and canola are suspected to cause tumor growth. Then I followed some advice from my friend Purvi Sevak and made a nice tahini and garlic dip for the cauliflower on the side. The recipe I found used yogurt, but I used coconut yogurt without much trouble. Since the point of the yogurt is to keep the cauliflower moist and to hold the marinade to together, you could probably even substitute coconut butter.

- 1 tablespoon coconut oil
- 1 head organic cauliflower
- 1 1/2 cups plain Greek yogurt/coconut yogurt/softened coconut butter
- 1 organic lime or lemon, zested and juiced
- 4 tablespoons tandoori marinade (i use Shan Masala but there are a number of brands that make it)
- 1 tablespoon crushed fresh garlic
- 2 teaspoons sea salt or himalayan salt

Preheat the oven to 400 degrees and lightly grease a small baking sheet with coconut oil. Set aside.

Trim the base of the cauliflower to remove any green leaves and the woody stem.

In a big bowl, combine the yogurt with the lime zest and juice, chile powder, cumin, garlic powder, curry powder, salt, and pepper.

Dunk the cauliflower into the bowl and use a brush or your hands to smear the marinade evenly over its surface. (Excess marinade can be stored in the refrigerator in an airtight container for up to three days and used with meat, fish, or other veggies.)

Place the cauliflower on the prepared baking sheet and roast until the surface is dry and lightly browned, 30 to 40 minutes. The marinade will make a crust on the surface of the cauliflower.

Let the cauliflower cool for 10 minutes before cutting it into wedges and serving it with a tahini dip or a nice raita (yogurt, mint, coriander, cucumber and roasted cumin seeds) and a salad.

Cauliflower Crust Pizza:

For the crust

- 1 large head cauliflower, chopped into florets
- 2 tablespoons of coconut flour
- 2 tablespoons of nutritional yeast
- 1 large egg (or 2 large tablespoons of chia seeds mixed with 6-8 tablespoons of water until the texture resembles raw eggs)
- 1 cup of freshly grated Parmesan or Asiago (or Daiya vegan cheese)

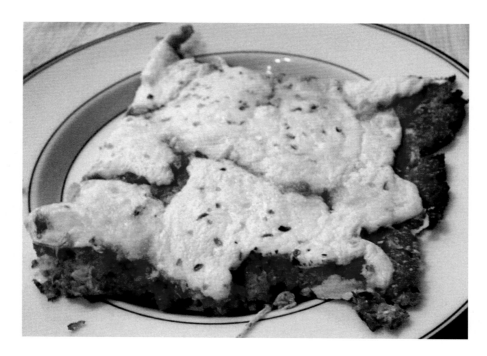

For the topping

- 1/2 cup crushed organic tomatoes with garlic and basil or organic pizza sauce
- 1 cup shredded mozzarella cheese (you can also use Daiya for the cheeses)
- 1/2 cup shredded cheddar cheese
- 1/4 cup fresh basil leaves
- 1/2 teaspoon crushed red pepper flakes, optional

Preheat oven to 400 degrees F. Line a baking sheet with parchment paper; set aside.

Start with the cauliflower crust:

Add cauliflower to the bowl of a food processor and pulse until finely ground, yielding about 2-3 cups. Or grate the florets, using a box grater. Add to a skillet and cook for about 10 minutes on medium heat so that it dries out and has flour consistency. Let it cool.

In a bowl, mix together the egg (or egg substitute) and grated hard cheese. Then mix in the cooled cauliflower. Sprinkle the coconut flour on top and then mix in.

Spread cauliflower mixture on the prepared baking sheet about 1/4 inch thick, thinner in the middle, thicker and more uniform on the sides so they don't burn. Bake for 19-20 minutes, or until golden. Let cool.

Topping:

Once the crust has cooled, swirl on the tomato sauce and the cheeses, drizzle with olive oil. Return to oven and bake until the cheese has melted, about 6-10 minutes.

Serve immediately, sprinkled with basil and red pepper flakes, if desired.

I recently made this with ground chia seeds for the egg (I am sensitive to eggs) and the teenagers ate it all up. If you're avoiding dairy, you can use daiya mozzarella in the place of the cheese. If you have a dehydrator, try drying out the cauliflower crust first, before baking

There are a lot more recipes in Joel Fuhrman's *Eat to Live* and Alexander Junger's *Clean Eats*—and even just looking online. When I eat raw—way easier in spring and summer—I like Organic Avenue or the Moon Juice cookbook. I WISH Karliin Brooks of The Squeeze would write one because her moc' n' cheese is worth going vegan for.

If it all feels like too much, there is an amazing organization called **Savor Health** that works with oncological nutritionists and finds the best diet for you. Then they prepare it and deliver it to you. They work alongside hospitals and doctors. Another delicious company is **Sakara** which creates organic, vegan and/or raw meals and delivers them to your door in the New York City area. Their websites are in the resources section. And there are many more, ask a friend to google organic, vegan, raw food restaurants and see if they deliver. Raw food has the advantage of helping your body cool and hydrate itself after the heat of the chemotherapy or radiation.

See? Not too hard! Start with one or two meals a day and then gradually ladder back!

If you fall off the wagon, do not stress. Have a bite or a taste of something you crave. Eat it slowly, enjoy it, savor it. They say we most appreciate the first and last bites of everything we eat. Two bites should be enough then. Eventually, your taste buds will be cleaner and you will find the taste of artificial colors and flavors will be harsh and chemically. Sugar will give you a sudden head rush and you'll discover how quickly grains bloat you and make you sleepy. It's ok to have a little from time to time. But let your body rest, too.

The most important thing is to take the time to believe that your food is made with love and prepared to nourish and heal you. Take the time to bless your food and feel gratitude for the planet and the Source which gives you food to eat.

Sometimes the belief alone will transform your food.

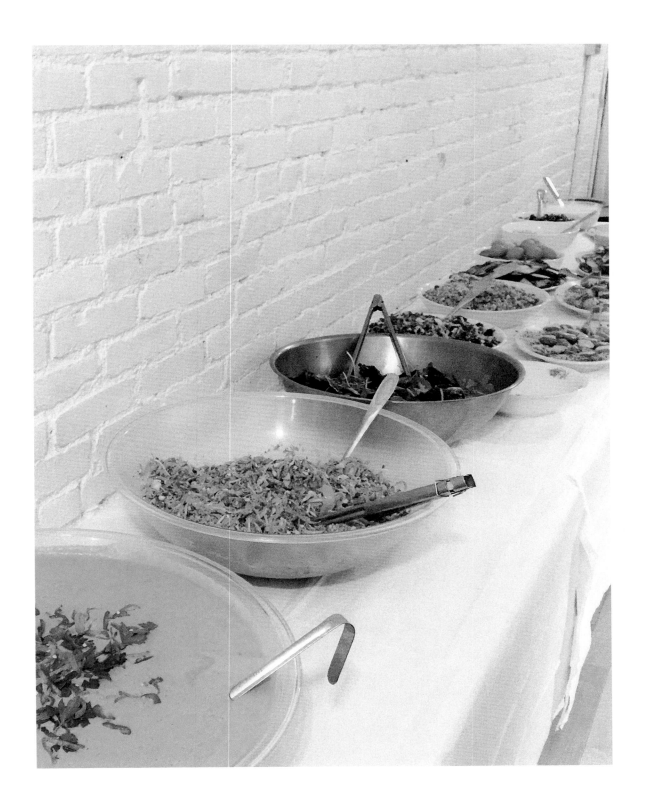

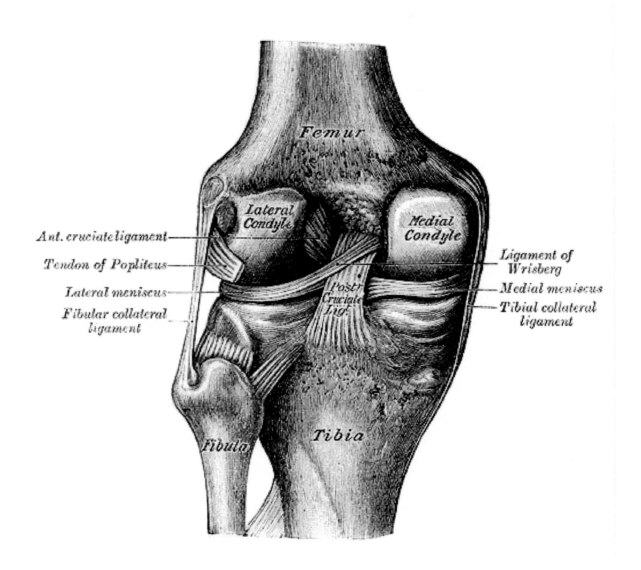

Femur

Lateral Condyle

Medial Condyle

Ant. cruciate ligament

Tendon of Popliteus

Lateral meniscus

Fibular collateral ligament

Ligament of Wrisberg

Medial meniscus

Tibial collateral ligament

Post. Cruciate Lig.

Fibula

Tibia

106

Feed Your Head

The Importance of Attitude and Energy Healing.

CHAPTER ELEVEN: Feed Your Head.

Energy work is essential to your treatment and survival. It changes how you feel and according to many of the modalities, a good energy worker allows your body to make the adjustments it needs to heal itself.

Once I was doing some energy work on my dad because the arthritis was acting up in his knees, I could feel the heat and activity in his joints in the palm of my hands so I asked him what he was experiencing.

He said, "I think I am imagining that I feel something." (I've told this story a million times because it made me laugh.)

My dad is a scientist and bases his opinions on physical evidence. I explained that from a purely quantitative scientific perspective, the reason one "feels" anything is because nerve receptors fire in the brain saying that there is pain or pleasure or cold or heat or anything in-between. So the reality is that anything one "perceives" is created in the brain. Thus when one takes a "pain-killer," it doesn't mean that the issue (the inflamed joint, stitches, spinal subluxations) is resolved, it just means that those nerve endings are numbed or quieted down. And one "imagines" that there is no pain.

There is a theory amongst health practitioners that all illness starts in the mind, or maybe in the metaphorical heart, if that is the seat of all emotions. The idea is that an emotional or psychological state is so unbalancing or upsetting that it gradually starts affecting the body. In Chinese medicine, there are esoteric explanations of illness along with the physical ones—lung issues may come from unresolved grief or may cause a sense of sadness, liver issues from anger, or an irritated liver may cause an irritable spirit, lower back pain from frustrated creativity, knee pain from fear, breast health from a woman's relationships or sense of herself as a sexual being. Obviously, my explanations are very general.

The simplest example is the tension headaches, TMJ, or neck and shoulder pain. While there may be a structural issue, it begins with feeling anxious or stressed and then clenching one's muscles.

To understand further, think about a dog or cat when they feel threatened. Involuntarily, they raise the skin and fur on the backs of their necks. Do that for a long time and the muscles get tired and pass the information on to the nerves—as an ache.

Thus many energy healers say, "The issues are in the tissues." While some people's worries settle in their scalps, others may be in their stomachs or spines. In *Oprah Magazine's* April 2014 issue, the article, "The Migraine in My Butt," by Juno Demelo, is about a woman who resolved the painful muscle deep in her glutes using meditation and soul searching for the issues behind it. Exploring the nonphysical side of her pain began with a book called *The Mindbody Prescription: Healing the Body, Healing the Pain* by a doctor who used to be the director of outpatient services at the Rusk Institute of Rehabilitation. Dr. Sarno's theories draw deeply from Freudian psychology and the idea that rage starts in early childhood, perhaps even in infancy, and can take over your life.

That's all very well to say.

Unfortunately, I've noticed that when someone with a chronic or systemic condition gets the suggestion that there might be a psychological or emotional aspect to it, they tend to get angry and offended: "Can you believe it? The doctor said it was all in my mind?!"

When a friend of mine who has an inexplicable, debilitating issue was told a hypnotist might help her, she was so insulted that she decided her doctor was an idiot.

So here's the thing:

The idea that an illness may be affected by your mind doesn't mean it's not real.

It doesn't mean your illness doesn't exist or isn't wrecking havoc through your body or your life. The idea is not reductive, patronizing, or dismissive. It doesn't mean the pain isn't keeping you up at night or making it impossible to do what you need to.

When an allopathic or Western medicine doctor suggests mind-body or energy therapies, it usually means that they don't understand how to resolve your symptoms. Why they don't understand may be for a multitude of reasons, they may be checking the wrong parts of your body, they may have missed a symptom, or it may be something else. It also doesn't mean that there isn't also a real external cause.

Almost everyone in healing has repeated the story of Dr. West and his cancer patient, Mr. Wright from the 1957 paper by psychologist, Dr Bruno Klopfer, "Psychological Variables in Human Cancer."

Mr. Wright had an advanced cancer called lymphosarcoma. All treatments had failed, and he wasn't expected to last a week. But Mr. Wright desperately wanted to live, and he heard about a promising new drug called Krebiozen that was being offered in clinical trials.

He begged Dr. West to treat him with the drug, but the trial was limited to people who had at least three months to live. Despite that, Mr. Wright was convinced that the drug would be his miracle cure. Eventually, Dr. West managed to obtain the drug and injected his patient with Krebiozen on a Friday. Dr. West assumed the man wouldn't last the weekend.

To his complete surprise, when Dr. West returned on Monday, his patient was up and around. Dr. Klopfer said, "The tumor masses had melted like snowballs on a hot stove," and were half their original size. Ten days later, Mr. Wright left the hospital, seemingly cancer-free. Then scientific literature reported that Krebiozen wasn't effective. Mr. Wright, who trusted what he read, became depressed, and the cancer returned.

So, Dr. West decided to try something. He told Mr. Wright that the initial drug had deteriorated during shipping, but that he had a new supply of highly concentrated, ultra-pure Krebiozen, guaranteed to work. Dr. West then injected Mr. Wright with distilled water. The tumors melted again, the fluid in his chest disappeared. Mr. Wright made a full recovery for another two months.

Unfortunately, the American Medical Association then announced that Krebiozen had proved utterly worthless. Upon hearing this, Mr. Wright lost all faith in his cure. His cancer returned and he died two days later.

So despite his recovery and relapse—his cancer was very real. The difference with cancer (and a lot of other systemic or chronic illnesses) is that the doctors often can't figure out the cause in order to eradicate it.

Think about it this way, if your mind and body are in balance, you can be exposed to bacteria or carcinogens and never develop any illness. That's why (as I've said before), someone can say, "My grandmother smoked five packs a day and lived on lard and sugar and died at 105."

That's also why someone who is physically addicted to cigarettes can be cured of their addiction using hypnosis. It doesn't mean there isn't a physical addiction, it just means that the mind is more powerful than you think (no pun intended). Lissa Rankin's book, *Mind Over Matter*, gives even more examples. For instance, a diabetic with a dissociative identity disorder whose other identity was not diabetic. Other people with dissociative identity disorder often have one identity who needs corrective glasses and one with perfect vision.

Following that logic, there is another—even more controversial—theory that I believe: Major illnesses (and major catastrophes) show up to heal your life.

There's an entire school of thought around this, including "an uncomfortable" book by another German doctor, Rudiger Dahlke, called *The Healing Power of Illness*. The idea is that quite often people dealing with chronic illnesses or pain have internal issues that they haven't had the time or space to resolve. When a crisis comes, it forces you to re-think.

It's almost a cliche that people who have cancer—or another brush with mortality—become much more sensitive to the simple pleasures of life. Certainly, being faced with death, puts the prosaic into perspective.

In my own personal experience, I've found that taking the time to be grateful for things, even horrid, painful, life-damaging things, opens me up in a new way.

If you are not well, or in a difficult situation, you might find this idea disgustingly Pollyanna, so I apologize in advance. but I ask that you just entertain the thought. Follow it through.

Usually, after I swim laps, I take a long shower (both terribly drying for the skin, I know) and find myself pondering my latest disaster and wondering what I have gained from it. I keep asking myself over and over again what benefit I enjoyed from being sick, being broke, being broken-hearted, or whatever loss or awful humiliation it is that time.

Usually, while I am drying off, I say to God or Universal Intelligence, "Thank you, thank you, thank you for letting me be here. Thank you for letting the water pipes break, because now I know that I need to remember to pay attention more to every day things. I need to look after them," or maybe "Thank you for the water pipes breaking because it is forcing me to fix the floors and I never would have done it."

(Apologies again for the pedestrian example, because that makes it seem easy.)

Perhaps doing this gives me an illusion of control, that events are not totally random, especially events inside my body. And perhaps it is a way of letting my mind open to healing. Because somehow, when I manage to reach the place of REALLY feeling grateful, everything starts shifting.

It does take me some time to get there, depending on how bad the situation is. I try to be grateful and instead, I am mad. I spend some time being compassionate with myself for whatever pain I am feeling. I tell myself there is a benefit and then I get mad at myself and say, "How stupid!! What could possibly be good about this?" I have to keep searching for the gratitude and keep exhaling the anger but eventually, it comes.

It sometimes takes days. Or weeks.

It is hard work.

And it doesn't mean you don't have to do the work of physically changing your habits, your diet, your responses.

You need to **GET HAPPY.**

People who are happier recover faster, live longer, and are more resilient. So what do you do if you are generally a darker person?

It seems that we are born with—or maybe develop in our very early lives—a happiness set-point. Like most of the stuff that is set in the very beginning (maybe even in utero), it's really hard to change.

Even more frustrating are all the people who urge, "Just be positive! It will all go well," when you know you are about the go over the edge of a waterfall in a rickety barrel. Or that's what it feels like. You're not being a pessimist, you're being a realist. For the record, telling someone, "be positive" is one of those uselessly irritating phrases like, "just calm down," "don't worry" or "just relax." Pain, fear and sadness are all real and valid feelings. The idea is not to pretend that they are not there or act like everything is great. Be ok with being sad or scared or hurting. If you gloss over it, you will feel worse.

The truth is, fear and suffering are great teachers and allies. You can work with them and get to another level. But you have be honest and ok with them being there. A friend of mine told me that in Japan they say, "Sadness is visiting me." It is a temporary state that you acknowledge without necessarily embodying.

Take the time to meditate, or "sit with," as they say in meditation circles, the pain, fear or sadness.

Because no matter what is happening, there IS a bright side of things. To return to the metaphor, maybe it's a really hot day and the waterfall is cool and refreshing. Maybe the barrel is watertight. Maybe thinking about that cheers you up a little.

Just the act of smiling—moving your lips into position—changes your endorphin response. So making yourself smile, when you're in a difficult position, can make you happier.

There is a way to get happy. It just requires work. Gretchen Rubin (of the Happiness Project) says that the one habit that almost all happy people share is making their beds in the morning. Perhaps it's just getting a sense of control over your life. It's doing something that makes everything look like it's in order. Whatever it is, it makes you feel happier.

Then another study showed that people who washed dishes were happier and felt less stress. Again, it's a simple chore that really changes how your kitchen looks. It's has a start and a finish.

But if you really want to be happier, wash someone else's dishes.

According to *Psychology Today*, studies show that the most effective way to change your happiness set point is to help other people. If you have cancer, your health could change drastically if you can make that shift.

There was a painful story in the New York Times magazine about a woman called Anna Lyndsey who is burned by even the slightest exposure to light. Her skin has become so photosensitive that she cannot even open the curtains during the day. While living in permanent darkness, she's written a memoir about it. At one point in the article, she warns against the "Lure of the Reiki Healer."

"Lyndsey writes of wanting, when the healer suggests that there is always some hidden benefit to being ill, to smash in the woman's face."

But the end of the article suggests something different:

"She describes the rainbow of colors she sees in the house depending on the weather outside, the various stages of dusk, the subtle differences between the light at sunrise and sunset. 'I went for a walk at dawn on Christmas day, which was the first time I'd managed to do that for years,' she said. 'It was absolutely deserted, and the sky was this lovely peachy, bluey gray, very tasteful, and there were all these magpies flying round the houses.' It's the kind of thing most of us see without seeing, a scene so ordinary it barely registers. sky, magpies, houses: nothing of note. for Lyndsey, rare and beautiful—art."

I don't mean to be reductive or dismissive. I can't imagine that experience. And it's possible that Lyndsey's beautiful walk was not a reward and, obviously, the physical reality of her illness is so much more than a metaphor.

That said, what makes sense to me and my experience of illness or catastrophe is that if you can understand what benefit you might gain from it, you can address the need that is not being satisfied and perhaps help your mind heal your body.

I had a similar conversation with the shrinks at Memorial Sloan Kettering. I explained why I no longer needed to have cancer. The psychiatrist was taken aback. "At Memorial Sloan Kettering, we don't believe cancer is a punishment!" He exclaimed.

Dahlke explains it better in the article:

"The problem is that people confuse responsibility and guilt," says Dahlke over Skype. "When I argue that someone is responsible for his illness, I'm not saying that that disease is his fault. The disease provides an ability to respond, however. We have to get to know what that disease means in our lives, what it wants to tell us. A disease presents a task, and when we perform the task, we heal the body."

If all life is experience created by perception and belief—and both of those things are created in the mind—couldn't changing the mind change the body?

We might even be able to create a new gene.

In my experience, approaching anything or anyone with love, understanding and acceptance always works better than anger, aggression or tension.

Just a thought.

Maybe you want to invite it in for a little while.

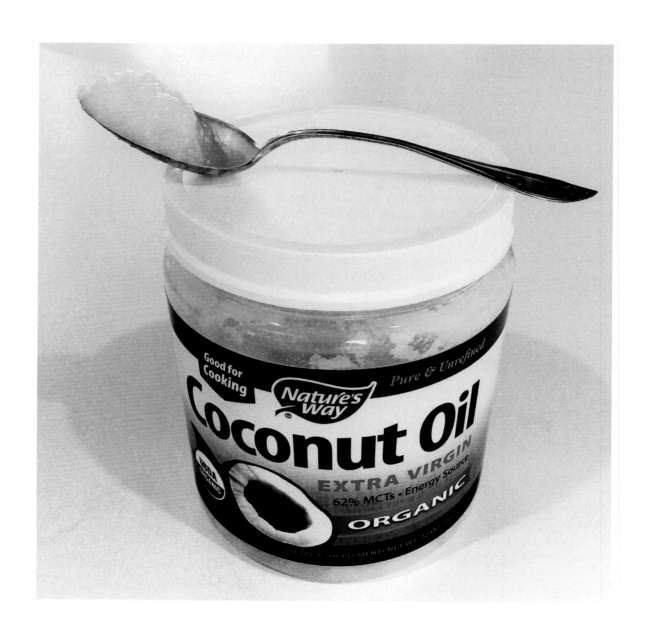

CHAPTER TWELVE

Can You Cure Your Cancer in 31 Days?

Ty Bollinger and the Truth About Cancer.

CHAPTER TWELVE: Cure Your Cancer in 30 Days.
Ty Bollinger and the Truth about Cancer.

This is the title of a book by Ty Bollinger, a regular person (a CPA, actually) who's done some incredible work on understanding cancer and alternative cures. Bollinger's film series, *The Truth About Cancer*, has interviews with some of the most interesting (and successful) voices in the alternative cancer care world.

Despite the confidence of the title and the fact that they sell it very hard online and that Ty Bollinger is a committed Christian and uses those metaphors in his work, the book actually has some very useful advice.

The question remains:

Can you cure your cancer in a month? I would say, yes. With some qualifiers:

1. How far your cancer has advanced.
2. How much chemo and/or radiation you've already had.
3. How much you are willing to commit to resolving it.
4. What kind of cancer you have.

People who have cancer call me about once a week with questions about what I did and how I did it.

So here are my own disclaimers:

1. I had a cancer that has a very high "cure" rate.

2. I did have 14 weeks of traditional EMACO protocol chemotherapy (though my experience made me believe that if my cancer were to return, I would never step into an oncology ward again. I stopped the chemotherapy before the tumor was gone and before I finished the course).

3. The symptoms—very heavy bleeding—made it easy to discover I had cancer. However, my cancer was extremely aggressive and fast-moving and (like lots of busy mothers) I ignored the hemorrhaging for six months.

I also swam laps—3/4 of a mile—daily, until the last month, and did Pilates every other day so it IS possible to be sick and not really realize it.

Personally, I recommend the book and all of Bollinger's work—not as the be-all and end-all—but because it addresses the physical parts of healing cancer very well.

Bollinger begins with the idea of the detox. I recommend a detoxification myself to **EVERYONE** who has cancer or any kind of degenerative illness—and then, a re-building of your strength.

1. **Eliminate sugars** (and anything that turns into simple sugar) from your diet. That includes wheat, white rice, potatoes, most fruit, corn—I sound like a broken record here. You might need to do this just until you are in remission, but maybe you'll feel so great that you want to do it forever—with the slight exception of fruit. You can start having more organic fruit once the cancer is resolved.

2. **Eliminate animal products**—many sources say that a cancer diet should be low-protein AND low-carbohydrate, especially during chemo. Listen to William Li's Ted Talk, "Can We Eat to Starve Cancer?" on youtube. Bump up cruciferous vegetables. Almost everyone knows that broccoli, kale, brussel sprouts, cauliflower, cabbage, and daikon (Japanese radish) are the enemy of cancer cells.

3. **Eliminate ALL processed foods.** If you have done the first two, you are probably forced to do this anyway. No artificial colors, sweeteners, nothing that comes wrapped in cellophane, no MSG, nothing from a fast food restaurant (where it is probably chemically-treated), no preservatives. If you can prepare your (organic) food at home—eat it fresh and quickly—you will always be better off.

4. **Heal your teeth.** Ty Bollinger—and many German doctors—suggest you address your teeth. First, like many naturopathic doctors, they suggest you get all your mercury fillings very carefully removed and replaced. Mercury leaches out from the fillings and damages your immune system. People who do this report having headaches and colds disappear. Next, there are a lot of illnesses lurking in the bacteria between your teeth and there is a theory that root canals—where a cavity exists inside your gum that is closed up and allows bacteria to hide and reproduce—can be the cause of everything from heart attacks to cancer. If you go to a holistic dentist, they can address the root canals as well as the mercury fillings using the proper materials so you are not exposed to the mercury. The idea behind the mercury removal is to strengthen your immune system to fight the cancer. At the time, I did not have the financial ability to do this. However, I did remove them recently and I found all my neck and shoulder pain disappeared instantly after the removal.

5. **The longer you've had cancer, the deeper its gone,** and the longer you've had chemotherapy and/or radiation, the longer your healing process will be. Simply put—and even doctors like mine at Memorial Sloan Kettering say—chemotherapy and radiation damage your "good" cells, your fast-growing cells (thus your hair falls out) and your immune system. Most forms of natural healing work by activating your own immune system in order to fight the cancer.

   Unfortunately, while you've been treating your cancer, you've been suppressing and damaging your body's own immune system.

   If your cancer is quite deeply entrenched, or you have had a lot of allopathic treatment, I suggest you learn to be very patient with your body.

   If you've ever been pregnant, you remember that the day after your baby is born, you are horrified to see that you still look pregnant. My midwife used to say "10 months up and 10 months down. (It's sort of the same way you recover from a bad relationship). Recovering from cancer takes time.

   Ty Bollinger suggests you start with a parasite cleanse. This takes about a week and can be done simultaneously with the liver and colon cleanse.

   In my classes in naturopathy and Chinese medicine, I've learned that almost all of us have parasites (some beneficial)—if you have ever eaten sushi, raw fruits and/or vegetables, and/or almost anything prepared in a restaurant, you probably have some malicious ones too. It doesn't take a trip to somewhere exotic to have parasites and they are often not obvious.

   The reason to kill the nasty parasites is to optimize your body's ability to utilize nutrients. It's not that hard as there are a number of kitchen plants and herbs that kill parasites, amongst the, ginger and garlic and oregano oil.

6. **After the parasite cleanse, the liver and colon cleanse help strengthen** your immune system and clear out the toxins that are building up from the chemo and/or radiation. I would recommend that everyone do a liver and colon cleanse, at least once a year. But if you are feeling very weak, these might be hard to do. You can find Hulda Clark or Andreas Moritz's versions online.

   For a gentler liver cleanse, my teacher of herbalism, Peeka Trinkle, suggests this. For 48 hours, avoid ALL fats, sugars (including fruit, potatoes, and alcohol), grains (wheat, rice, oats, barley, quinoa), caffeine, and animal products (no meat or dairy), no medicine (not even aspirin or tylenol, which settles in the liver)—with NO CHEATING, not even a teensy bit. Lots of well-meaning people say, "just a little bit won't hurt..." In this case, it will—don't do it.

   Drink at least three liters of water a day and as many fresh vegetables as you can eat. If you can handle it, drink a spoonful of organic apple cider vinegar in water every few hours.

This detox has been known to get homeless alcoholics to get over the alcohol sickness and dry up for a little while.

After a liver cleanse, you'll notice immediately that your skin is brighter, the whites of your eyes clearer and the bags under your eyes depuff or disappear entirely.

7. **Eat a ketogenic diet.** Check **Chapter Ten.**

8. **Since Bollinger is a Christian, he suggests you go to church.** I suggest you increase your level of prayer and/or meditation, wherever you do it—at church, a mosque, a synagogue, a temple, forest, or beach—to help you manage stress, tension, and anxiety.

9. **Add anti-tumor supplements and foods to your diet**—including large amounts of turmeric, quercetin, vitamin C (pure l-ascorbic acid), vitamin D3, bitter almonds, cesium chloride, potassium, Essaic tea, co-Q 10, and Polymva. (I am not suggesting you rush out and fill your shopping cart. Work with a good naturopath or natural pharmacist to get your dosage and brands. I recommend speaking to David Restrepo at Vitahealth in NYC, they deliver all over the country.

10. **Take probiotics in the morning** and pancreatic enzymes with every meal.

11. **Make sure you get a lot of sleep**, at least eight hours a day—if possible, 10.

12. **Drink only purified water**—chlorine and fluoride are carcinogens—you need to avoid them at all costs.

13. **If you are strong enough to exercise, do it.** Walk, do yoga, Pilates, swim (in non-chlorinated water), bicycle, run, or lift weights if you can. It doesn't have to be intense, but it reduces your chance of cancer by 50% and increases your chance of recovery.

In reference to my own exploration of alternative and complementary medicine, someone asked me how I figured out which things to do. How did I know which were scams? "How did you decide?"

Me: "I just did everything non-invasive that anyone suggested."

That's not completely true. Everything that I read or heard about or that was suggested to me, I investigated online and with friends to see if there was real back-up. I also checked if it had more than one source that recommended it. I cross-referenced it with the crucial database www.cancertutor.com.

How to Cure Your Cancer in 31 Days is somewhat similar in that its program addresses the physical cancer from every angle.

Like Bollinger, I agree, there is NO SINGLE CURE. It's not just acupuncture, hypnosis, getting enough vitamin D3, or juicing, or even switching to a total raw diet will work on their own if you don't address all the cleaning and strengthening—and even more so, if you don't address your mental and spiritual state.

Anxiety, self-doubt, and tension will take you down, my friend.

In the end, if you are strong and committed enough to actually follow all the recommendations in Bollinger's book, I believe you WILL cure your physical cancer in a month.

In the meantime, download or buy the DVDs of the The Truth About Cancer. You will be inspired.

However, the cancer could come back if you ignore your mind and your programming. Personally, I'd recommend working with a good hypnotist and/or an energy healer to help calm and activate your subconscious and improve your self-talk.

Be well.
You can do it.

It just takes work and a real commitment.

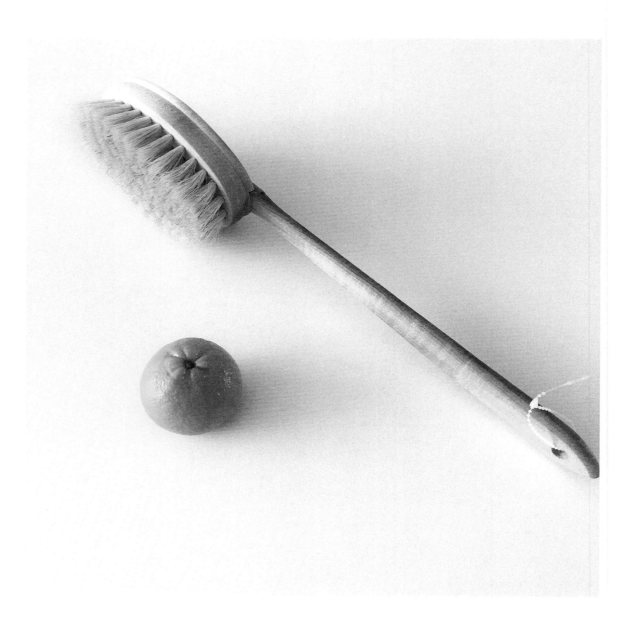

Dry brushing or body brushing can smooth away orange peel skin and help heal cancer.

Bouncing, Brushing and Lymph.

Why jumping up and down and dry-brushing is so important.

CHAPTER THIRTEEN: Bouncing, Body Brushing, and Your Lymph System

If you have cancer—or almost any chronic illness—you owe it to yourself to try body-brushing. It's a cheap, simple way to make your skin and lymph nodes more effective at eliminating toxins and producing vitamin D3. Your skin is your body's largest organ and, when working properly, eliminates 25% of the toxins in your body every day. In natural medicine, your skin is called your "second kidney" for its importance in clearing fluids and wastes from your body.

If you are simply a healthy person, it also strengthens your immune system, increases circulation, reduces cellulite, smooths away stretch marks, gets rid of ingrown hairs and blocked pores, and exfoliates for the softest, baby skin you ever felt. The other benefit is that many people find the process meditative, restorative, and energizing, all in one.

Think of it this way, any dead or dry skin cells on the surface of the skin block the healthy ones from light and oxygen so it's harder for your skin to produce the vitamin D it needs to keep you healthy. Also, by stimulating the skin, you stimulate the lymph system, which is a highly-sensitive series of tiny tubes that lie just beneath the surface of the epidermis, transporting waste from your tissues to your blood for elimination. When your lymph system is inflamed or blocked, you are more likely to develop disease.

Start like this — go to your local health food store or bath and body place or amazon or thrive market—and a buy a natural fiber body brush. Mine tend to cost between $6 and $12 and last about a year. It is should be firm and a bit scratchy-feeling. NOT TOO STIFF because the idea is not to rub yourself raw. For your first body brush, I'd suggest one that is slightly softer so you ease into it.

In the morning, before the shower, strip down and start brushing at your feet. Remember this is DRY brushing. Do it before you are wet. No oils or products on your skin, it's just you and the brush. The idea is to always brush towards your heart, from bottom to top. Brush each foot, top and bottom, from the toe to the top of the foot and up your leg to your thigh. Stop there and brush the other leg.

Then brush the abdomen. Personally, I follow the direction of the colon to also help with my digestion. If you do a search online, you'll see amazing before and after pictures of loose or puffy tummy skin being tightened up with regular brushing. Brush briskly so that your skin feels stimulated but not irritated. You can get a long-handled brush for your back.

Some people suggest brushing in small circles around your joints to loosen the fascia and release tension and toxins there.

If you have bad acne, I've read suggestions of a soft brush for the face—and seen incredible before and after images, but I have never tried it. You would need to wash your brush with soap and water regularly to avoid spreading bacteria.

Take a shower after the brushing and massage your skin with sweet almond oil as that helps soothe and heal the skin. Then apply any body lotion or product you like (but try to stay away from the junk, no matter how good it smells). You've just strengthened the moisture barrier on your skin so you're pretty protected now.

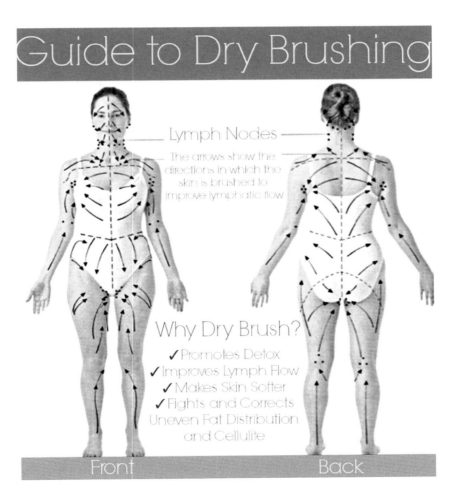

So what about the bounce?

If you are getting chemotherapy or radiation, your skin may be too sensitive for brushing. Mine felt thin and irritated all the time. Chinese medicine practitioners suggest using a rebounder—or a simple mini-trampoline—to keep the lymphatic drainage going.

This is equally easy and simple. You get on it once or twice a day and bounce gently for 10 minutes, more if you feel like it. You don't need to get really vigorous, it's not gymnastics. If your balance is off or you feel shaky, you can put the rebounder next to the sofa or a heavy piece of furniture to hold on to, or buy one with a handle. Shift your weight from one leg to the other and you will also help increase your bone density and improve your balance.

The motion of your body also helps stimulate the lymphatic system. I've read accounts of people with lymphoma who incorporate rebounding along with juicing and avoiding sugar and animal products who have had lumps and tumors resolve themselves with no other intervention. It's worth a try.

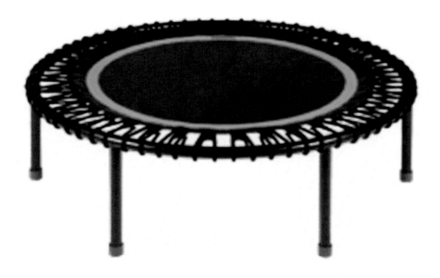

Daily rebounding can also be useful for cancer patients.

If you want to get fancy, try a Powerplate or another vibration platform. Many gyms and spas and even, chiropractor's offices have them. Just standing on one of these machines for two to four minutes, twice a day, not only stimulates the lymph, it strengthens your muscles and increases your bone density which is very useful when aging, chemotherapy, or radiation can make your bones porous.

Cancer especially seems to affect the lymph system—whether it's lymphoma, breast cancer, or thyroid cancer—so any or all of these are worth adding to your healing or protective arsenal.

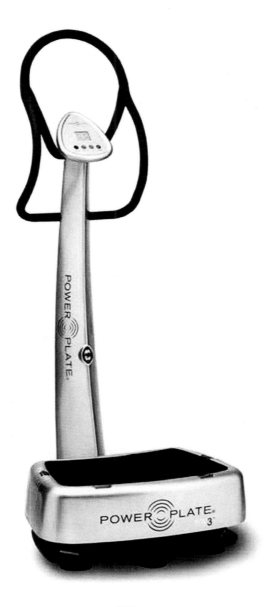

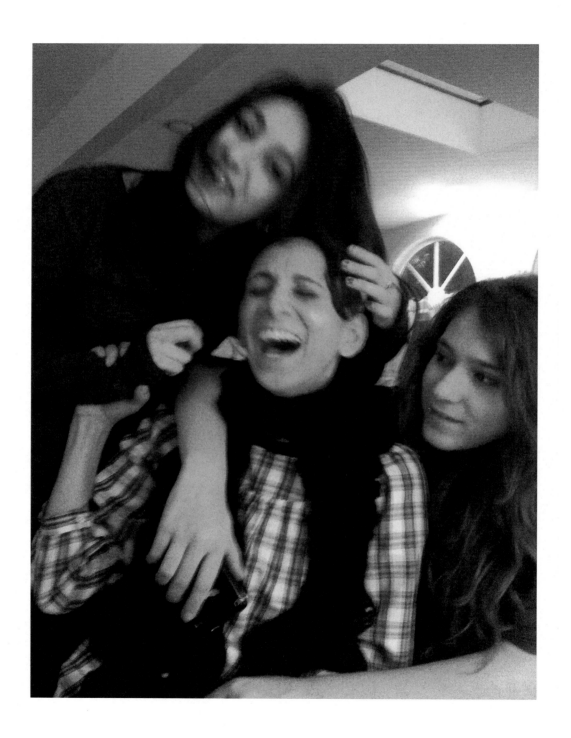

Friends, Family and other Challenges.

Dealing with the people who love you – and practical advice for friends of cancer patients.

CHAPTER FOURTEEN: Friends, Family, and Other Challenges

One of my most vivid cancer memories is checking my cell phone midway through a chemotherapy session and seeing a text from my friend and upstairs neighbor, Purvi Sevak: "Your kids seem to be having a party."

When faced with a parent-free home on the weekend, what would most teenagers do? (There are lots of movies to answer that question.)

When I was first diagnosed with cancer, my teenagers were on the cusp of adolescent fever. Sasha was 16, but gentle, caring, and cautious. Zarina was just 13 and wearing the array of party dresses she'd accumulated for her year of bar and bat mitzvahs. Jahanara was nine and babied by her older sisters. (Fortunately, she was at her father's house that night.)

The party went on to be a complete bust. They smuggled in a six-pack of Mike's Hard Lemonade (a small amount of vodka watered down with sugary lemonade). One young friend knocked back a fifth of vodka and collapsed on the floor, which had the slightly positive result of adults barging in to get him to a doctor and breaking it all up.

That was just the beginning. All the teenagers spun out of control for a little while. They were so angry and frightened and desperately attached to me at the same time.

The point of this story is that when you get cancer, the reactions of the people around you are completely unpredictable.

Just when you most need your kids to be dependable, they act out. When you need your parents or aunts and uncles to love you unconditionally, they point out the reasons (they believe) you got cancer in the first place. Some friends rise beautifully to the occasion, some acquaintances turn into confidants, some are cruel, some vanish.

I address two audiences here...

1. You are a person currently has cancer or some other debilitating illness or

2. You are a friend or family member of a person (I hope just one at a time) struggling with cancer or other debilitating illness or circumstance.

ONE, You're in it. You're the cancer survivor.

Yes, it's intense, probably the most overwhelming experience in your life. It's hard not to be cross with your friends when they get to get up and walk out of the hospital room back to real life.

They get to wash their hands, leave, and get a coffee on the corner or get in the car and drive home. Their bodies don't ache and they can move their arms and legs comfortably and eat everything they want without feeling sick.

What I was most envious of my friends when I was sick was their control over their lives. All those choices and options. When you are really sick, you end up having to hand over your autonomy. It's like being a baby. Most of the time, you are grateful for the help. But sometimes, you just want to get up and make your own dinner just the way you like it. Sometimes, you are sick of the way your caretaker makes a stir fry every single night because she can't think of what else to do with all the vegetables you need to eat.

Here's what you need to do:

Remember, people **WANT** to help you. Be gentle with them.

1. When someone asks if they can help, give them specific tasks.

An Errand—"Would you mind stopping at the organic grocery and getting me fresh turmeric root or some dark chocolate?"

A Meal—Ask them to cook or bring you something you are dying to eat. To avoid disappointment, be clear: "I can't eat dairy," or "I hate okra," or "Thyme is my least favorite herb" (those are all my issues). Or be even more specific, point them in the direction of a recipe or restaurant you like.

Babysitting—Take your kids shoe shopping or out to lunch or the movies. Sometimes, when their parent is sick, the home can feel oppressive. Kids need light and air. It's good to get them out and laughing. Tell your friend not to get all heavy with them.

Organizing—Personally, I LOVE people to come and open my mail and throw away all the junk and file all the bills, or put all the books in the bookshelf properly. Or open the cupboards in the kitchen and put the plates and bowls in order. I love it even more if they don't make comments about my sloppiness or financial insolvency at the same time.

Phone Calls— If a friend can't come visit or is too faraway, you could ask them to make calls for you. Maybe ask them to return a bunch of phone messages, or help you research something, or call your dry cleaner or the electric company or anywhere you can't (or you're too tired to) email.

Any of these are so much more useful and less expensive than a half-wilted bunch of flowers from the supermarket.

2. Don't get irritated when no one does things the way you want.

Everyone is frightened and trying to do the best they can. Actually, this is good advice any time anyone who loves you does something for you. If you are a control freak like me or you are feeling anxious while you are sick, this is very hard to do.

Sometimes your ex-husband is going to buy them shoes that are highly impractical, your boyfriend is going to forget the organic coconut water, your mum is going to cook the broccoli 'til its soggy, your friend is going to bring you ginger rather than turmeric root, and you just have to say, "Thank you."

Because they all deserve acknowledgement and love for their efforts. And just because they do things differently, doesn't mean that they do things wrong.

In other words, maybe you really NEEDED ginger (very good for nausea) and you didn't realize it.

Breathe. Be grateful.

3. Be loving with the friends and family members who disappear. Or behave badly.

One of my amazons said, "I hope you get cancer all over your body and die." Some of my closest friends never came to see me or dropped off the face of the earth.

It is scary. So incredibly scary to watch someone you really care about getting very weak or thin or losing their hair. If the sick person is one's parent, imagine how scary it is to lose the person who is meant to look after you, especially when you are not ready for it.

Remember that everyone is processing information in their own way. We are all in different stages of evolution. You never know what is happening in your friend's personal life, or what happened in his/hers personal history that is activated by your illness.

Your illness is a difficult circumstance. The person's reaction now doesn't negate any of your history. And it probably means that he or she still loves you, she just has her own stuff to cope with.

If your friend or family member uses the opportunity of your cancer to "punish" you for some perceived mistakes in your life, remember that he is doing that because he's invested in you in some way.

Breathe. It's all about love and fear.

You need to use the former to get over the latter.

That can mean faith—choose whichever one speaks to you—use Love or God or Universal Intelligence to focus on the bigger picture, to put it all into perspective. In my case, it meant Sufi chanting, repeating the name of God endlessly on a string of beads.

Try and stay connected to the Source. That energy coursing through you will help you be transcendent. Don't get pulled down into anyone else's struggle.

Day-to-day anxiety and tension is part of the reason you got sick to begin with. So if they start to get to you, fly away. Even if it's just in spirit.

Keep breathing.

TWO, you are a friend or family member.

1. Please come and visit.

Especially in the hospital during chemotherapy. Chemotherapy, for most people, means sitting for hours or days in a chair or a bed with an I.V. attached to your arm. The chemo drugs burn terribly as they go in. Sometimes it makes you dizzy or nauseated or cold. If you are near enough to spare an hour or two, please come and tell the person jokes while they are confined. It can get lonely and tedious.

Sometimes, the person getting chemo can't see properly, so don't bring anything too complicated, but a silly video on an iPad or a laptop is great. Or come and sit beside the person and distract them with funny stories or gossip. If you're really stuck, get some of those stupid celebrity magazines they have in the nail salon. You can laugh about Kim Kardashian's outfit or speculate on whether Jessica Chastain is jealous of Jennifer Lawrence, anything superficial and idiotic is a relief.

In the hospital, one lies there waiting for their insipid meals, so it's wonderful to have someone come to hang out with you. Maybe bring something fun from outside, like slipper socks to wear from the bed to the bathroom. Or a really nice organic hand lotion or a box of organic blueberries.

2. Please be flexible and patient.

When one gets home from chemo, one feels horrid. It's exhausting and painful. One just wants to get into one's own bed and lie quietly. No conversation. I liked company on my up days, but I also had lots to do because I only had three days a week when I could walk around outside and not feel awful or drained.

So what I mean is—try to find out which days are better for visiting. Maybe email or text your friend or his/her caretaker to get a sense of the rhythm of things.

If you come over and your friend isn't there, drop off your gift or card and don't get your feelings hurt. Or if you come over and your friend just doesn't feel like seeing someone, just come another time.

When you come to someone's home, don't stay for too long. Your friend gets tired easily. Leave before you notice her/him fading.

3. Don't telephone.

Personally, I found it really difficult to talk on the phone. It made me dizzy and nauseated. I am not sure if all people undergoing chemo have that reaction, but if the electromagnetic rays from cellphones are still being questioned, why add one more thing?

On other hand, if the person has a normal landline, maybe he/she likes talking on the phone. I didn't mind it in hospital at all.

4. Come over and help.

Ask if you can take the kids out for the afternoon, do a load of laundry, wash the dishes in the sink.

Ask, but don't ask too much. It's embarrassing to ask for help, even if you are weak and sick. Just look around and see what needs to be done. Maybe ask if you could sort out the books in the bookshelf (see above) or fold and organize all the sheets and towels in the linen closet.

You could check if the apartment has all the basics, like cooking foil and plastic wrap (necessary evils), napkins, toilet paper and paper towels, eggs, milk—whatever the regular stuff is—and replenish and put away the stuff that's missing.

Maybe you can help with some bookkeeping or cook dinner (just don't leave a gourmet-sized stack of pots and pans and double-boilers).

5. Listen

Whatever you do, remember that the person who is sick has lost some control over his/her life. Try and help your friend or family member get some back. He/she might be irritable or very picky about how he/she wants things. It's not just general unreasonableness, it's frustration.

So ask your friend what she wants and follow the instructions no matter how ridiculous.

Let your friend vent. Yes, of course, there are people in the world who have it worse. You might have great ideas for your friend. But unless, he/she expresses an interest in those ideas, don't push it.

6. Make them smile.

If your friend is now bald and weighs 80 pounds, common wisdom says don't comment on their appearance. Personally, I preferred people being honest. The jokes about being hairless or looking like a space monkey or whatever cheered me up.

I felt like, at least they said what they were REALLY thinking. When someone said, "Oh my gosh, you look great!" I never trusted them again. Unless, the friend qualified it by telling me how much better I looked since I started juicing or acupuncture or whatever.

Laughter is great for your immune system, even NIH has posted studies about it. Just like in the hospital, tell your friend funny stories. Bring really silly DVDs—though be careful you don't offend their sensibilities. Since my brain was working at half-speed, I needed to watch idiotic stuff. I used to love witticisms. After chemo, I liked slapstick.

7. Pay a Bill

Many people facing cancer in the U.S. are overwhelmed by the costs. They are probably not working during the time of their treatment and much isn't covered by insurance – if they have and can afford insurance.

8. Whatever you do, stay in touch.

If all you can do is call, call. If you stop by to visit and she's out for a walk, just leave a note. It makes a difference, having people around you helps you heal faster and better. Don't let your friend feel like she's in it alone.

9. It's not over 'til it's really over.

It can take a long time to recover from cancer. You have to recover physically, emotionally, socially, financially.

Be gentle.

Your friend can probably use a bit of extra support for some time. If you missed the chemo/radiation treatment part, you still have a couple of years to make up for it.

Love and Cancer

Staying married
or not during a crisis.
Dating while bald
(is not as bad as you think it is).

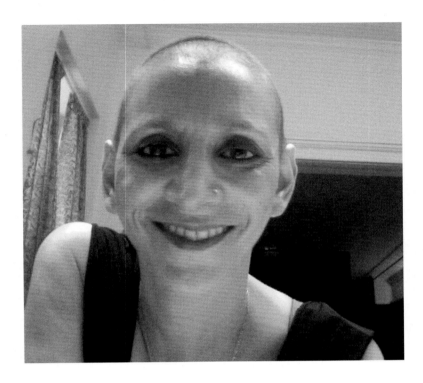

CHAPTER FIFTEEN: Love and Cancer

I was at a book reading recently, chatting up an editor about my cancer book. I explained the near impossibility of finding new love when one is undergoing cancer treatments.

She told me about a novel that everyone was talking about called *[SIC]*, written by Joshua Cody. What she found fascinating, she said, was that he was so interested in sex. His book is a raunchy and musical ride through his romantic and occasionally drug-addled adventures whilst undergoing a very difficult treatment.

I found myself both cowed by the beauty and poetry of his writing and shocked by the sheer nakedness of it. He writes about his experiences vividly.

He sneers at the pastel-covered cancer memoir genre: diagnosis, realization that life is wonderful, and eventually moving to a little cabin in Vermont. His is a dangerous, vicious, thrilling book.

But I find myself relating. If nothing else, when you are single when you have cancer, you long to have someone chronicle the transformation of your body. In the same way that when you are pregnant, your body bloats and ripens and turns into another beast entirely, your body when you have cancer, morphs and betrays your expectations again.

It is both frightening and beautiful, in the way that a Francis Bacon painting is—a beautiful ode to the human form, even in its most grotesque condition. While having chemo, one's skin turns pale. At times blue, at times, mottled with red spots. The flesh seems to fall off the bones. And the bones, those bones, become so sharp and apparent. You lose your hair — that means ALL your hair, on every inch of your body. There is something alien about the body so hairless, fleshless and pale, I wanted pictures to explore the strangeness.

In my case, my fingers and tongue took on a blackish tint, as if stained with ink. I had tiny, burning sores on my cheeks and wide swaths of little blisters on my ribs, like stripes. I think about the woman in the cancer support group in the movie, *Fight Club*. Bald and wasting away, she was dying to find a one-night stand before she left the world. When I first attempted the occasional date again, not long after I stopped treatment, a guy told me I reminded him of her. I protested, I was so restrained — but the desperation and loneliness must have been obvious.

My cheeks and eyes were sunken and my lashless eyelids were burning and swollen. My eyes stayed bloodshot for months afterwards. While I didn't approach anyone, I longed for a warm body in the bed beside me. To be held and kissed by a being still surging with life, still pliant with flesh. I felt like a succubus, yearning to feel someone else's life force inside me.

Perhaps, though, because I refused the steroids and tried to keep up with Pilates, I never had the adrenaline-fueled energy to roam the streets at night or to go to parties and bars, like the character in *[SIC]*. I generally was in bed by nine, usually with Rara, who was just 10 years old and frightened, wrapped around me like a scarf and my mother sleeping fitfully on the sofa, a few feet away.

And then of course, there is the movie *50/50*. That very funny Seth Rogan comedy about a young guy (played Joseph Gordon-Levitt) who gets cancer. Since his insane girlfriend cheats on him, he is forced to go to bars with his buddy who uses his friend's cancer as a pick-up line.

This is where the cancer experience of women and men parts ways. The line, as everyone knows, would bomb. Basically, women (not all, but most) are hardwired to want to take care of people. A woman will sleep with a man because she feels sorry for him. A man? Not often.

There were a few guys who'd chased me over the years. When I got back in touch and mentioned the cancer—just a temporary state, I explained—I never heard from them again.

The statistics are something like this: three out of four men leave their wives/partners within a year of their cancer diagnosis. A woman is six times more likely to be separated or divorced after a cancer or MS diagnosis.

While the narrator in *[SIC]* had an encounter with a fellow cancer patient, she was an exmodel. And even then, she didn't come looking out great.

For the most part, if you are a woman, telling a potential suitor you have cancer (or even HAD cancer) is akin to telling him you're a leper.

Add to that three fashion-fascist daughters, very involved parents, complicated ex-husbands, and the disastrous ruins of my financial life post-cancer and mid-recession. Almost anyone I met—even online—would run screaming in the other direction.

I did have one date, not long after the chemo finished. I did my best to ice my eyes and tried to use make-up to make up for the pallor and lack of hair, eyebrows, and eyelashes. Upon shaking my boney hand, he looked pale himself. He tried to squirm out so quickly. He had barely received his order before he looked at cellphone and remembered another appointment in Williamsburg that he was already late for.

Perhaps that's why I watched the first season of *The Big C* with such satisfaction. Laura Linney chose to simply live with her cancer. She chose to enjoy the languid pleasures of summer without disclosing it and live as if every day was her last. And Idris Elba is a dream. Luckily for her, her cancer moved slowly enough to allow her to drag it out.

Perhaps that's why, only months after I finished treatments, I fell head over heels for a sweet 27-year-old who made me feel beautiful just four months post-chemo. I am still grateful to him for bringing me back to life. We started as friends online—though my suggestion is to simply meet people around you – open up to the world as you come back into it.

No house in Vermont yet. Despite that, I am still hopeful and optimistic that if the time is right and you are ready, you'll meet someone.

CHAPTER SIXTEEN

Staying Solvent While You Are Sick.

Facing your finances is crucial.

CHAPTER SIXTEEN: Staying Solvent When You Are Sick

I've read a ton of books on treating and surviving cancer, interviewed 30 people who've survived cancer using alternative methods, a wealth of healers who have assisted people using western protocols or worked with people who chose to opt out.

But no one's ever mentioned money. Or how to deal with your finances when you are sick. Or, the harder one, I think—how to deal with your finances when you come out the other end.

"Bankruptcy rates among cancer patients are nearly **2X** higher than the general population"

If you are sick, here is crucial advice. **PAY ATTENTION TO YOUR FINANCES**. In the new age world, we say, things grow when they have attention. It's like a houseplant, if you water it and put it in the sun, it will grow. You don't have to have the answers, you just have to see what's what. (I admit that this is not my strength). Just start.

Talk to your doctor about the cost of your care. Only 19% of people do—because they are scared they won't get such good care. But the truth is, your doctor may be able to help

141

reduce some of the costs, especially if you don't have insurance. I spoke to a doctor recently who told me that they often work with patients—and sometimes reduce the cost up to 75% depending on what they can afford. I have friends who have negotiated with the billing departments of hospitals and managed to get their bills down 50 to 75% or more. It should not reduce the quality of your care at all.

The other thing I recently learned is that if your doctor is doing blood tests or labs, find out where he/she is sending them. The labs charge you separately and they are also willing to help you out, especially if your doctor is already making concessions. Try calling the lab and asking if they can get you the results for less. If they can't, ask the doctor—sometimes different labs and diagnostic centers—even right across the street from each other charge totally different prices. Again, another friend found out the lab where her son's blood was being sent was very expensive. She asked someone in billing at the hospital and was told to walk across the street. The first lab was charging $1300 for the results, the place across the street—which was not as pretty, admittedly, but just as accurate—was charging $350.

One of my friends said, "You should spend whatever it takes to heal your cancer, because what good will your money do you if you are dead?"

This is true. But if you live, what will you do if you can't afford it any more?

Unlike standard chemotherapy, radiation, and surgery, which are generally covered by your health insurance, alternative care requires you to pay out of pocket right from the start. (One could argue that, if your health declines having chemotherapy, you will end having greater costs in the long run. Most insurance, brutally, will only cover you up to a point. But that's another story.)

On the other hand, if you are self-employed or you lose your job while you are sick, you will need to clean up the financial tangle when you get well. In the current economy, that can take some time, so be patient with yourself. For me, it was useful to remember that having a lot of money doesn't make you a better person—or more of a success—though it may feel that way.

After a lot of leg work, I found two very kind financial advisors from Forest Hills Financial Group who gave me some insights. Daniel Hochler and Isaac Cohen both had experience with family members with cancer and other illnesses so they know how difficult it is to face both things at the same time. They will actually come to your home and try and make sense of your various bank accounts, insurance policies and debts.

Of course, the first piece of advice is what everyone hears—the best way to prevent a financial collapse when you have a major illness—is to have at least a years' worth living expenses of saved. Plan ahead. Sadly, that doesn't work for many people.

My advice is—the minute you are diagnosed—you, and a friend who isn't judgmental, go through all of your paperwork and get an overview of your finances. (I mentioned lying in bed, waving to a paper bag full of unopened bills and crumpled receipts, and Isaac did say that was not the best way to start. So organize what you can, in a way that makes sense.)

You may be pleasantly surprised to see that when you get the big picture, it's not all that bad. Perhaps you have very little debt. Or perhaps you do have a lot of debt, but you have assets that you could liquidate (or sell). Isaac suggests that you look at every possible asset you have.

When I was diagnosed, I had already been out of work for several months and my savings were gone.

So here are some things you can do, even when it feels like you have no options.

1. Life Insurance—Do you have permanent (not term) life insurance? What Isaac told me is that you may be able to sell the policy. You may also be able to take out a loan against it. Check to see if your insurance has disability coverage or long-term care coverage.

2. Retirement Savings and 401(k)—Do you have either of these? Again, you may be able to either withdraw some or all of it, or take a loan against them.

3. Mortgage, Credit Cards and Car Loans—Call them and tell them what's going on. A lot of banks will actually give you a "forbearance," which means that your loan payments are deferred for some time. While this actually doesn't do you a lot of good, it does take the pressure off. If you can afford to keep your payments up, I suggest you do it, because when the forbearance period ends, you will suddenly have a lot on your plate again. But do call your banks and credit cards and tell them you are sick or recovering and they may be able to work with you. It's when you don't call them back that they start going a bit crazy. Also, keep records of all your phone calls—get the names of who you spoke to and when—just in case they don't keep their side of the bargain. You'd be surprised, with credit cards and car loans, you may have some negotiating room to lower your interest rate or find a lower pay-off amount.

4. Get a Little Help From Your Friends. I know a number of people who've used **Youcaring** or other crowd funding sources to cover some of their extra expenses. There is a crowdsourcing especially for cancer patients called **GiveForward**. They have good advice, but I don't know if they have the reach of an **IndieGoGo**. I was also amazed at how many of my friends gave me gift cards to **WholeFoods** or organic restaurants. What is good is to get a friend who can be an intermediary so that when people call or email or Facebook to ask how they can help, your friend can ask them to help pay a bill or donate a gift card to a juice bar or a grocery store.'.

5. Credit Rating—Make sure you look at this thing. It seems scary, but it's worth checking regularly when you are not well, because you don't know if there are any discrepancies. If you have a friend who wants to help, ask them to sit beside you on the bed and read things aloud to you. If there are discrepancies, your friend could write a letter on your behalf to correct them.

6. Get Friends to Help You Contact These Resources for Cancer Patients The only hard thing is that when you are not well or recovering, a cordless phone, or a computer screen can make you feel sicker. So see if you have a healthy friend who can help you make the calls.

7. Cut Back Where You Can—The minute you are diagnosed, find ways to trim your budget. Personally, I cancelled my newspaper subscription and reduced my cable to the minimum. I took my car out of the parking lot and parked on the street. I don't go to Starbucks anyway so that wasn't a problem. But find ways to cut back that won't affect your emotional state (remember, you need to feel good so you will get well). Buy your household supplies in bulk—send a friend to Costco or Sam's Club. Send another friend to the farmer's market for fruits and vegetables. Eat home rather than eating out—which is wiser when your immune system is compromised.

8. Don't Cut Back On the Stuff You NEED for Your Health—Even your emotional health. If that means juice, acupuncture, energy work, and organic food, try to find the best way to get that stuff. Especially if you are still weak.

9. Get a Financial Advisor—If you have a bit of money saved, think about having someone advise you on the best way to organize your assets so that you will not come back to total devastation when you are well. BEWARE there are people who work for big insurance companies who call themselves financial advisors when they are really salesmen. They will sign you up for annuities that have exorbitant fees if you try to take out the money in less than 10 years. I worked with a manipulative "friend" called Lesley Edwards who worked for Mass Mutual and probably made an enormous amount of money off me by convincing me to put all my investments under his control. It cost me a lot of stress and money to get any of it back.

10. Your Home—Unless you have a lot of help, I wouldn't recommend selling your home while you are ill or in recovery. You need a sanctuary and a safe place to be. If you have a place that you could move to, effortlessly, and people to help you in the process, that is another way to free some cash. If you live in an expensive rental—and again, you have help—you might move to a cheaper one. But this is really a last resort if you are not well.

11. Look at your car and homeowner's and other insurance. You might be able to greatly reduce your monthly premium payments by raising the deductible (this is what you would have to pay out-of-pocket if you have an accident, before the insurance payments kick in).

12. Wills and Trusts—It's a good idea, early in your treatment, to make sure you have a will and everything in it is the way you want it. My suggestion is to do this not immediately after being diagnosed—when you are still in a panic and not thinking clearly—but once the details of your treatment have been decided and you have a little rhythm. You don't want to do it late in the treatment, because, especially if you are doing a conventional treatment, it can make you weak and too tired to think. Also, remember that the computer emits an EMF that is theorized to slow healing, so don't spend too much time on it when you are weak.

I had left everything I owned to my daughters, who were, at that point, minors. What Isaac explained is that if I had passed away, everything would actually have gone to their fathers who were their adult next-of-kin. He told me that lots of divorced people did not want to leave their homes and property to their exes! Instead, he suggested I create a trust for the girls. Today, I would leave everything to Sasha who is 23. Knowing that she is a very caring older sister, I would leave her to divide the assets with her younger sisters.

Issac reminded me that in the midst of the chaos, one needs to remember the kids. Make sure that they know that there is a plan in place so they will be looked after. If they are old enough to understand, get them involved in the financial planning, but don't make minors beneficiaries, because then their adult guardians will make the decisions for them.

If you run a business, create a transfer strategy to make sure your family is protected, no matter who your successor is. Review the ownership of the business and separate your assets.

Though once you get well, that's when things get really tough. At that point, your creditors and family members are often exhausted of trying to help you hold things together.

And in this economy, it's tough to pick up the pieces.

One idea is to contact **Debtors Anonymous**. They are all over the U.S. and can help you not do what I did, which is not look at anything and hope that it would go away.

They have regular meetings and can help you organize the way you face your creditors.

In my case, in desperation, I called 311. They directed me to an NYC program called the **Financial Empowerment Center**. A bright young woman called Elena actually looked through all my paperwork and created a spreadsheet with my monthly income and my costs. She also looked through my credit rating with me and helped me correct errors.

She recommended lawyers and tax accountants who did pro-bono work. Apparently, this is a nationwide initiative that is expanding. So if you are in the U.S., try contacting them.

However, BE CAREFUL OF PAID CREDIT COUNSELORS! There are lots of unsavory ones who make money off you and/or steal your identity and other horrid things. Try and find a government-initiated program or get a referral from a friend.

Just remember that money is not scary (I tell myself this), it is energy and numbers. Don't give it power over you. Like your body, it needs you to pay attention to it to stay healthy.

If you can survive a major illness, you can survive a major financial setback. Lots of people come back even stronger.

If you are a friend of a person recovering from an illness, offer to help with that stuff. You have no idea how long it takes to get back to normal.

And keep breathing. You will get there.

Breaking Up With Cancer.

Life-threatening illnesses
actually have a bright side.
Get ready to let go.

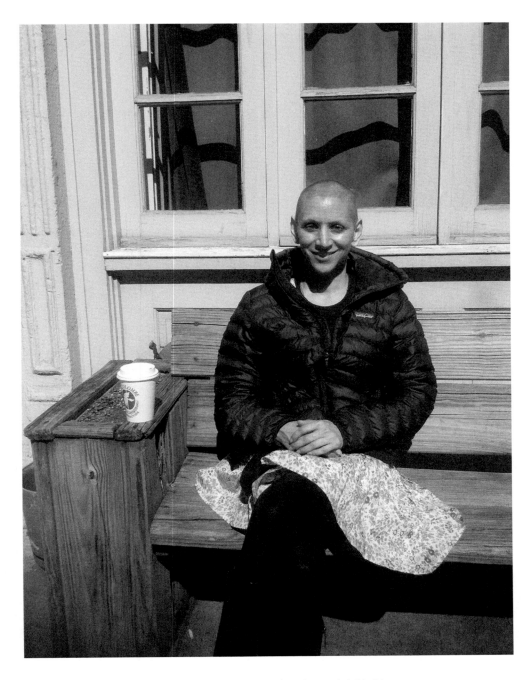

Let's face it, having cancer does have a bright side.

CHAPTER SEVENTEEN: Breaking Up With Cancer

Let's face it, having cancer does have a bright side.

People let you skip to the front of the line at the bathroom or in a crowded theater. They might give you tickets to a sold-out show. Give you a free meal on the restaurant.

When you call your bank and tell them your mortgage or credit card payment is late because you have cancer and you're getting treatments and you can't work, they might be really nice. They often reduce fees or eliminate them. They say they won't report your late payments.

Friends bring you presents or invite you to events. You get an all-access free pass to all kinds of stuff. You get a great excuse. You can leave an event early, space out on someone's name, say something stupid. You can take a nap at any time of the day and no one thinks you the worse for it. When you go out to dinner with people, they always want to pay for your meal.

If you struggled with your weight before, you might have the pleasure of being extremely slim. You can wear clothes that never fit you before. Before I was diagnosed, I was eating four peanut butter and jam sandwiches a day, along with regular meals, and still losing weight. (Admittedly, it can go from supermodel gaunt to emaciated very quickly. Making that "you can never be too rich or too thin" pillow, whether it was Babe Paley or Wallis Simpson's, a lie.)

Your kids can skip school occasionally or not do their homework. Everyone gets let off the hook. There is a bright side to contracting one of the most feared illnesses in modern history.

If you are starting to bounce back, if you feel your body and spirit respond to the work you are doing, you have to make a painful choice.

This is quite possibly the hardest thing to face in your recovery process. It's when you make the decision to let go of your cancer. When you decide that you will no longer be a sick person. When you won't let anyone take care of you any more.

If you've gotten this far, you're saying, "OF COURSE, I WANT TO LET IT GO! Are you a total idiot?"

There was a guy who read a story at the Moth about recovering from a life-threatening accident and what happens when you decide to take ownership of your life again—it's a shock. You might not be prepared to hit the pavement quite so fast. The banks aren't nice any more, even if you don't have a job yet.

It can take you a long time to recover from such a massive change in your financial, emotional and physical being, but when you decide to take that step, it's like being born again. That can be harsh. Think about it—cold, naked, and disoriented. What makes it even harder is that, unlike a newborn, you are not starting with a blank slate. It's like coming home from vacation. No one else finished all the work that was piling up on your desk while you were gone. You just have to do it.

When you have a doctor's appointment, no one comes with you any more. People stop sending you flowers. When you get a phone call or a letter, you just have to deal with it yourself.

Remember that thing about washing dishes? You have this huge pile in front of you and the only way out is to roll up your sleeves—maybe put on your rubber gloves—and get on with it. If you leave everything a bit of mess, or expect it to all fall back into place, you will be judged harshly for it.

WHAT IF?

Even more scary—you could get well just to lose everything. Maybe your boyfriend or girlfriend or husband or wife left or will leave you in your process. It's an intense journey and maybe the other person couldn't handle it.

Maybe you couldn't manage your bills and you are on the verge of losing your home or getting your car repossessed. Why get well if you're going to have to face a material reality that is so hard? Isn't easier to stay sick and in a little bubble where people are loving towards you and give you a break?

In a way, having cancer can be its own reward. People might reward you by forgiving you for anything you did in the past. They are kind in a way you don't feel like you deserve.

Or maybe being sick helped open up a part of you that you didn't know was there before. It can be an opportunity to re-visit places in yourself where you were hurt or hurt other people. It can be a chance to re-think stuff about yourself you don't like.

That's why it's so hard to stop being a person with cancer. It's also so much easier to just "follow the protocol" that the doctors give you. You leave the illness to someone else and you let it happen.

Last of all, in the United States at least, dying is considered the ultimate failure. Medical care failed if you die, you gave up the fight if you die. When I decided not to have any more chemo, a friend, said, "What's wrong with you, Ameena? You have kids! You have to fight it!"

I said, "I'm not willing to fight death and give up my life. What kind of life would I have if I was sick from all the treatments? I might be alive but what kind of life would I have? And how would that be good for my kids?"

If you are reading this book for a friend, or if you've just come across this chapter by mistake, I suggest you read one of the many books written about death and the afterlife. If you've had enough, death is just the next step in the journey. It may be that you feel like you're ready for closure.

BUT YOU'RE NOT DEAD!

Invest in your life. That includes meditation, meeting up with friends, exercising, eating food that nourishes you. A friend of mine is writing a great book on survival after an illness. Because, from what I can see, there is no instruction book on what you need to do to keep thriving afterwards.

After I had my first kid, in London in 1993, I found a book called *The Next Nine Months: A Guide to Your Body After Giving Birth* by Paula M. Siegel. It was the only book that I have read to this day that addresses what happens to your body and soul in the months AFTER you give birth. What's interesting is that there are all these books and websites about being pregnant and having a healthy baby and all these books about dealing with a baby and a toddler, but it seems like—after you give birth—they drop you like a hot potato and move on to the kid. No one talks about how to deal with episiotomy scars or tears or headaches from epidurals or how it feels to no longer own your body.

So, when you are ready to break up with being sick, make sure that everything you do is an investment in being well. For instance, instead of thinking about a wardrobe for the hospital, think of what you can wear to work out. Think about what you can do to give yourself more vitality and more support for being healthy and whole.

If you are struggling, this is a great moment to go to a hypnotist and get a session. You will come away with affirmations designed especially for you and a greater awareness of your blocks. If your hypnotist is good, she or he will give you an MP3 or a recording of your session so you can listen to it while you fall asleep at night.

This is a great moment to see a therapist so that you can complain and give yourself compassion for the struggle you are going through. It's good to have a person who can help you face your limitations and give you the moral support to get through them.

I suggest you fire your caretakers, too. I had to tell everyone to leave and stop holding my hand. That way I had to take care of myself and get myself in order. My polarity and craniosacral therapy teacher, Gary Strauss, used to say, "Time to put on your big girl panties."

It's hard and when you are ready, you can do it.

Take a deep breath. Take it slow. Take it easy.

But let it go.

You'll be great.

Resources:

CHAPTER ONE:

U.S. Cancer Report
www.cancer.gov/research/progress/annual-report-nation

Mitchell Gaynor
www.newsmax.com/Newsfront/mitchell-gaynor-nyc-natural-health-doctor-deaths/2015/09/17/id/692115/

Chlorine and Cancer
www.seeker.com/chlorinated-pools-may-increase-cancer- risk-1765106407.html

Otto Warburg
www.nytimes.com/2016/05/15/magazine/warburg-effect-an-old-idea-revived-starve-cancer-to-death.html?_r=1

CHAPTER TWO:

Sprout Growing Kits
sproutpeople.org/raw-food/

Alkaline Drops for your water
alkazone.com/wpcproduct/mineraldrop/

Heat Therapy
www.cancer.gov/about-cancer/treatment/types/surgery/hyperthermia-fact-sheet.
http://drsircus.com/medicine/light-heat/hyperthermia-far-infrared-cancer-pain

Bio-Mats
www.bio-mats.com/far-infrared-studies#cancer

Pranayama Breathing
www.mindbodygreen.com/0-4802/3-Powerful-Pranayama-Breathing-Exercises.html
www.artofliving.org/us-en/yoga/breathing-techniques/alternate-nostril-breathing-nadi-shodhan

Essiac Tea
amazonsofnyc.blogspot.com/2013/11/the-c-word-essaic-tea.html

Frankincense and Myrhh
http://drericz.com/frankincense-oil-cancer-immunity/
https://thetruthaboutcancer.com/frankincense-and-cancer/

ENERGY HEALERS

Penney Leyshon
www.penneyleyshon.com/

Maha Rose Collective
www.maharose.com/

POLARITY THERAPISTS

Ellen Kruger
http://soma-psycheinstitute.com/02-ellen.htm

Gary Strauss
Life Energy Institute

BRENNAN HEALING SCIENCE

Laura Styler
www.awakenyourpower.com

ACUPUNCTURISTS

Mona Chopra
www.peopletreewellness.com/Mona/Welcome.html

Ming Jin
www.drmingqi.com/about/about.php?pg=3

Dorene Hyman
www.dorenehyman.com/Dorene_Hyman/Welcome.html

Maryam Mehrjui
www.heartbodymindacu.com/

HOLISTIC NUTRITIONISTS

Eileen Cuce
www.eileencuce.com

AROMATHERAPISTS

Donna Shepper
www.lighteob.com/

RECONNECTIVE HEALING

Peter Goldbeck
http://edgarcaycenyc.org/index.php/are-teachers-a-group-leaders/157-peter-goldbeck

BEAUTY ADVICE

Mary Schook, Beauty Engineer
www.beautybymaryschook.com/

HOMEOPATHS

Peeka Trenkle
www.peekatrenkle.com

Susan Sonz
www.wholehealthnow.com/bios/susan-sonz.html

HYPNOTIST

Tracy Beers
http://hypnosischangeslives.com/

MASSAGE THERAPIST

Charles Michener
http://bcmassage.amtamembers.com/

CHAPTER THREE:

HPP processing
http://dailyburn.com/life/health/the-truth-about-hpp-juice-labels

JUICE RECIPES

Kris Carr, Crazy Sexy Cancer
http://kriscarr.com/crazysexyjuicebook/

Joe Cross, Fat, Sick and Nearly Dead
www.rebootwithjoe.com/recipes/

Broccoli Sprouts
http://pages.jh.edu/~jhumag/0408web/talalay.html
www.mercola.com/article/diet/broccoli_sprouts.htm

Ty Bollinger
https://thetruthaboutcancer.com/

Josef Issels
http://issels.com/publication-library/issels-holistic-integrative-approach-to-cancer/
#sthash.SbmZpnmL.dpbs

Oil Pulling
http://amazonsofnyc.blogspot.com/2016/05/the-c-word-oil-pulling-or-running-pipes.html
www.healingcancernaturally.com/detoxification-oil-pulling.html#how-to-instructions-for-oil-pulling

DIETS

Alejandro Junger
www.cleanprogram.com/

Fred Bisci
www.yourhealthyjourney.org/

Norman Walker
www.myhdiet.com/healthnews/rev-malkmus/norman-w-walker-juicing-pioneer/
https://en.wikipedia.org/wiki/Norman_W._Walker

Max Gerson
http://gerson.org/gerpress/dr-max-gerson/

David Wolfe
www.davidwolfe.com/category/health-longevity/food/

Cancer Tutor Diet
www.cancertutor.com/cancer-diet/

Doctors and Standing Up for Yourself
http://content.healthaffairs.org/content/27/5/1416.full.
www.bestdoctors.com/

Elle Woods in Legally Blond
www.youtube.com/watch?v=vO5gXBF559I

CHAPTER FOUR

Robotic Surgery
www.hopkinsmedicine.org/news/media/releases/hospitals_misleading_patients_about_
benefits_of_robotic_surgery_study_suggests

Information on Hysterectomies
www.hersfoundation.com/facts.html

Cancer Ads Use More Emotion Than Fact
www.nytimes.com/2009/12/19/health/19cancerads.html

How to Choose Where to Get Your Cancer Care
www.nytimes.com/2009/12/19/health/19cancerside.html?action=click&content
Collection=Health&module=RelatedCoverage&region=Marginalia&pgtype=article

Diptyque
www.diptyqueparis.com/home-fragrances/scented-ovals.html

Brad's Kale Chips (and other snacks)
https://bradsplantbased.com/shop/crunchy-kale/crunchy-kale-nasty-hot-6-pack/

Natural Wipes and Sanitizers
http://herbanessentials.com/
www.eoproducts.com/

CHAPTER FIVE

Happier People Heal Faster
www.sciencedaily.com/releases/2010/08/100802101622.htm

Weleda
http://usa.weleda.com/our-products/shop/calendula-face-cream.aspx

California Baby
www.californiababy.com/creams.html

Liquid Gold Radical C and Cell Quench
www.cellquench.com/

Cleopatra's Cream
http://priestessalchemy.com/html/cleopatra_skincare.html

Illuminare Chemo-safe Make-Up
www.illuminarecosmetics.com/product_p/c-260.htm

Hashmi Kajal
www.hashmisurma.com/hashmi_kajal_stick.html

Mary Schook, Beauty Engineer
www.beautybymaryschook.com/

Ameena applies false eyelashes
www.youtube.com/watch?v=4LvYyk7FDS8

Fasting During Chemo and Radiation
www.scientificamerican.com/article/fasting-might-boost-chemo/
www.sciencedaily.com/releases/2016/07/160711150926.htm
www.hope4cancer.com/information/healing-cancer-on-time-how-intermittent-fasting-may-
help.html
www.myhealthwire.com/news/breakthroughs/924

Natural Fragrance Oils and Body products
www.floracopeia.com/
www.naturopathica.com/

Meg Cohen's Cashmere Hats
www.megcohendesign.com/

CHAPTER SIX

Is Your Doctor Being Paid by Pharmaceutical Companies?
www.propublica.org/series/dollars-for-docs

Does Your Doctor Work Too Many Hours?
http://nymag.com/scienceofus/2016/03/why-are-some-doctors-arguing-for-a-return-to-dangerous-exhausting-work-hours.html

Pharmaceutical Companies Falsifying Research
www.businessinsider.com/pharmaceutical-firms-accused-of-falsifying-data-in-major-alzheimers-study-2014-1
www.cchrint.org/2013/04/08/be-skeptical-of-pharmaceutical-company-claims/

What Doctors Don't Know
www.ted.com/talks/ben_goldacre_what_doctors_don_t_know_about_the_drugs_they_prescribe

CHAPTER SEVEN

Dr. Mitchell Gaynor
www.gaynorwellness.com/about-gaynor-wellness/
www.nytimes.com/2015/09/20/health/mitchell-l-gaynor-59-manhattan-oncologist-and-advocate-for-alternative-treatments-dies.html

Vitahealth Pharmacy and David Restrepo
https://vitahealthblog.wordpress.com/tag/david-restrepo/

Galina Semynova, Acupuncturist, Chinese Medicine
www.vitalgate.com/about

Dr. Oz's Five Supplements
www.doctoroz.com/slideshow/vitamin-essentials?gallery=true).

Nicholas Gonzalez
www.dr-gonzalez.com/history_of_treatment.htm

Vitamin D3 and Soy
www.inspire.com/groups/advanced-breast-cancer/discussion/the-latest-news-concerning-vitamin-d3-shocker-to-me/
www.thecancerguys.org/2013/01/soybean-oil-one-of-most-harmful.html
www.stopkillingmykids.com/why-you-should-avoid-soybean-oil/

Delgado Protocol for supplements
www.delgadonaturals.com/all-products-1/

Dried Herbs
www.mountainroseherbs.com
www.flowerpower.net/

Supplements
www.luckyvitamin.com
www.purencapsulations.com
www.revgenetics.com
www.vitahealthrx.com

Hippocrates Institute for re-setting your life
http://hippocratesinst.org/

Post-Radiation Bath
www.whydontyoutrythis.com/2013/12/sea-salt-and-baking-soda-best-all-natural-remedy-for-curing-radiation-exposure-and-cancer.html

CHAPTER EIGHT

PolyMVA
www.polymva.com

Cancer survivor testimonials
www.youtube.com/watch?v=KonHb6Q7MOE

Gary Matson interviewed by Walter Davis
www.youtube.com/watch?v=-1IT46YXtqo

Co-Q 10
www.epic4health.com/

CHAPTER NINE

Thich Nhat Hanh Foundation
www.thichnhathanhfoundation.org/?gclid=CM2q_OPxxdECFYiLswodco0N4g

Essiac Tea
www.youtube.com/watch?v=NhmeeguXPV4
http://essiacinfo.org/caisse.html
www.amazon.com/Essiac-International-500-veggie-caps/dp/B0016KJA0Y/ref=pd_sim_hpc_3)
www.amazon.com/Flora-Essence-Herbal-Blend-Liquid/dp/B0010EG6IK/ref=sr_1_8?s=hpc&ie=UTF8&qid=1383840374&sr=1-8&keywords=essiac%2Btea&th=1. It

Burdock
www.naturalnews.com/031524_burdock_root_herbal_remedy.html
www.women-info.com/en/fibroids-natural-remedies/

Slippery Elm
www.centerforhomeopathy.com/slippery-elm/

Sheep Sorrel
www.wildmanstevebrill.com/plants.html
www.anniesremedy.com/herb_detail468.php

Turkey Rhubarb
www.mountainroseherbs.com/products/turkey-rhubarb-root-powder/profile

CHAPTER TEN

Ketogenic Diet
www.cbn.com/cbnnews/healthscience/2012/December/Starving-Cancer-Ketogenic-Diet-a-Key-to-Recovery

Joel Fuhrman
www.drfuhrman.com/shop?gclid=CICdsLibx9ECFROBswod_FYBcQ

Dr. Mercola
www.mercola.com

Paul Pitchford
http://healingwithwholefoods.com/

Real Salt
http://drsircus.com/salt/real-salt-celtic-salt-and-himalayan-salt/

Omega VRT 350 Vegetable Juicer
www.omegajuicers.com/vert350-juicer.html
www.youtube.com/watch?v=q7mYHYuGu-g

Juice Shops
https://juicepress.com/
www.juicegeneration.com/
http://thesqueezejuice.com/

Mercola Probiotics
http://probiotics.mercola.com/

Cancer-fighting Meals Delivered
http://savorhealth.com/
www.sakara.com/

CHAPTER ELEVEN

Changing Your Happiness Set-Point
www.psychologytoday.com/blog/happiness-in-world/201304/how-reset-your-happiness-set-point

The Girl in the Dark
http://tmagazine.blogs.nytimes.com/2015/02/03/anna-lyndsey-girl-in-the-dark/?_r=0

CHAPTER TWELVE

The 31 Day Home Cancer Cure by Ty Bollinger
www.cancertutor.com/cancer_treatments/
www.amazon.com/31-Day-Home-Cancer-Cure/dp/1450799736/
ref=sr_1_4?ie=UTF8&qid=1484578833&sr=8-4&keywords=ty+bollinger

The Truth About Cancer
https://thetruthaboutcancer.com/

Parasite Detox
www.naturalnews.com/037964_parasites_detox_cleanse.html

Idelle Brand, Holistic Dentist
www.thebrandwellnesscenter.com/

Ketogenic Diet
http://articles.mercola.com/sites/articles/archive/2013/06/16/ketogenic-diet-benefits.aspx

David Restrepo at Vitahealth
www.vitahealthrx.com/retailer/store_templates/shell_id_1.asp?storeID=
B09DDEC26F1D4FB788C88A5316C0E904

William Li – Can We Eat to Starve Cancer
www.ted.com/talks/william_li

Liver Cleanse
www.curezone.org/cleanse/liver/huldas_recipe.asp

CHAPTER THIRTEEN

Body Brush
https://thrivemarket.com/

Rebounding Benefits
https://wellnessmama.com/13915/rebounding-benefits/

Bellicon Rebounder
www.bellicon.com/us_en/benefits/health-benefits/lymph-and-edema?gclid=
CJiE8IKBx9ECFY-NswodDFkHYA

Powerplate
http://powerplate.mercola.com/faqs.aspx
www.hypervibe.com/us/blog/7-whole-body-vibration-moves-for-improved-
lymphatic-drainage/

CHAPTER FIFTEEN

Love and Cancer
www.telegraph.co.uk/culture/film/starsandstories/8824832/Joseph-Gordon-
Levitt-How-I-made-cancer-funny.html
www.sciencedaily.com/releases/2009/11/091110105401.html
www.politicsdaily.com/2009/05/07/marriage-and-cancer-a-fairy-tale-it-aint/

CHAPTER SIXTEEN

Talk to Your Doctor About The Costs
http://blogs.webmd.com/cancer/2013/05/talking-to-your-doctor-about-financial-concerns.
html
www.newswise.com/articles/view/603148/?sc=mwtr&xy=5022899

Forest Hills Financial Group
www.fhfg.com/

Financial Resources for Cancer Care
www.cancercare.org/publications/62-sources_of_financial_assistance

How to Use Your Life Insurance
www.fifthseasonfinancial.com/

Crowdfunding for Healthcare
www.nbcnews.com/health/cancer/crowdfunding-cancer-care-how-more-are-covering-
costs-n368386
www.crowdcrux.com/tips-crowdfunding-medical-bills-expenses/
www.youcaring.com/
www.gofundme.com/medical-fundraising
www.giveforward.com/p/cancer-fundraising
www.indiegogo.com/

Financial Empowerment Centers
www1.nyc.gov/site/dca/consumers/get-free-financial-counseling.page
http://cfefund.org/

Debtors Anonymous Counseling
www.debtorsanonymous.com

CHAPTER SEVENTEEN

Gary Strauss, Polarity and Craniosacral Therapist
www.eomega.org/workshops/teachers/gary-b-strauss
https://lifeenergyinstitute.net/gary-strauss/

Made in the USA
Middletown, DE
17 February 2017